"Jeanne Magagna displays a rare combination of psychoanalytic rigour firmly based in infant observation, combined with a deep knowledge and experience of working with other modalities and disciplines, in order to understand and treat the complexity of children and adolescents with eating disorders and their families. Her compassion for the young people's suffering shines through in the many case examples, showing the therapeutic perseverance needed as well as a strong belief in the rightful need of these children for a container to process their emotional experiences sometimes for the first time. She emphasises the early infantile and primitive anxieties at the core of these children's suffering. She shows the resources needed to help these children and their families to bear these anxieties. This valuable book is for professionals working with this client group as well as with the parents who suffer the torments of living with such an unforgiving illness."

Ricky Emanuel B.Sc. M.Sc. MACP MBPC, Consultant Child,
Adolescent and Adult Psychotherapist, Teacher and Supervisor –
Tavistock Clinic London, Birmingham Trust for Psychoanalytic
Psychotherapy, Centro Studi Martha Harris, Florence

"With her wealth of experience as a practitioner and a teacher Jeanne Magagna deals with difficult patients who are prone to self-harm and suicide. Her innate ability to connect to them and their parents with kindness, gentleness and clear thought frees the anorectic young person's vulnerable self. Her honest and open clinical accounts go beyond recognizing the patient's projections to being genuinely affected by them, and then working through her own countertransference experiences. The most satisfactory therapeutic outcome is achieved when parents are helped through parents' groups, couple therapy and family therapy to work with the children to repair broken connections. A worldwide must-read for professionals, parents and young people, particularly those concerned about eating disorders."

Micky Bhatia, Child Analyst and Training and Supervisory
Analyst, Indian Psychoanalytical Society

"What happens when the relationship to the internalised parents is too conflictual and anxieties cannot be contained emotionally? At some point, either during childhood or adolescence, severe eating disorder may appear, along with the threat of death. Jeanne Magagna brings us close to this complex and desolate emotional territory, plagued with nightmares, feelings of persecution, and degrees of retreats so severe that language fails. She describes her clinical approach in detail, based on the establishment of a sensitive individual therapeutic relationship, the analysis of transference and countertransference, and belief in the beauty and goodness of the mother, her mind, her body, and her interiority. By building a container for those primitive terrors which were never contained, and enhancing the containing function of the parents, the multidisciplinary team arrives at emotional understanding and recovery of the children and their families. Beautiful task, beautiful book."

Mónica Cardenal, Training Analyst, Psychoanalytic Association of Buenos Aires. COCAP IPA, Child and Adolescent Psychoanalysis Committee Co-Chair Latin America. Supervisor in the Early Childhood Area and Director of Infant Observation post graduate Course, according to Mrs. Bick's method, Tavistock Clinic model, Pediatric Mental Health Service, Italian Hospital. Co-editor with Jeanne Magagna of **Revista Internacional de Observación de Bebés,** *Gradiva, Peru (2018)*

"This important book flows from many years of experience, written by one of the leading psychotherapists in the field of eating disorders. Magagna's extensive knowledge, her compassion and insightful wisdom are woven throughout its pages. She guides the reader though the work of communicating with distressed young people and exploring their emotional experience and the nature of our relationships and interactions with them, always focussed on enhancing therapeutic understanding. Numerous clinical examples bring these themes to life and will resonate with anyone working with young people with eating disorders. The writing is open, honest and reflective throughout. This text will appeal to all therapists – irrespective of training, professional discipline, or theoretical persuasion – interested in opening their minds, and seeking to improve their own understanding of the young people with whom they work. In this way Magagna indeed allows the door to be opened a little wider for countless emotionally imprisoned young people to be able to take those vital steps forward towards release."

Rachel Bryant-Waugh, BSc, MSc, DPhil, FAED, Consultant Clinical Psychologist and Lead Clinician ARFID Service, Maudsley Centre for Child and Adolescent Eating Disorder, London, UK

"Jeanne Magagna shares with us her many years' expertise in working with young people who suffer severely, and with the families and the caretakers committed to helping them decide to live. Jeanne emphasizes the therapist's empathy in bearing their hatred, disregard, being closed out from children who cannot trust, who are depressed, suicidal, in a claustrum, catatonic or suffering hallucinations. With detailed, close-in clinical examples, Jeanne shows how she works in the countertransference as a way to understand her patients' suffering. Read the book from beginning to end! You will feel fortified to move forward in your own work. You will be moved! Jeanne's closing remarks about her own emotional growth in working with these children will leave you teary-eyed and grateful."

Nancy Bakalar, MD, FABP, Supervising Analyst, IIPT, Chevy Chase, MD and Faculty, Denver Institute for Psychoanalysis, Denver, Colorado

"Reading Magagna's book on releasing the imprisoned self is like sitting in a library with an old friend, taking you on a journey from the very earliest stages of development of the child's mind, describing various ways in which this can go off course and develop into one form of an eating disorder or another. Interweaving rich observational and clinical material with theoretical illuminations drawn from the writings of leading psychoanalytic minds, Jeanne Magagna breathes meaning and hope into the therapist's mind to deal with young people who are often terribly hard to reach and help.

This publication offers a treasure trove of compassionate insights into the minds of people with eating disorders, particularly those with anorexia nervosa. The insights will resonate with and illuminate not only the clinician familiar with psychoanalytic ways of working, but all clinicians dealing with young people with eating disorders and their families, addressing common challenges that make these conditions some of the most difficult to treat."
Jeremy Freeman, Clinical Psychologist, Psychoanalytic Psychotherapist and Development Director, Australia & New Zealand Academy for Eating Disorders

A Psychotherapeutic Understanding of Eating Disorders in Children and Young People

This important book shows how psychotherapy can address severe eating disorders in children and young people, illustrating the ways an imprisoned self can be released from suffering.

The book features a range of case studies while addressing core issues such as self-harm, hallucinations and the threat of suicide, as well as related topics such as depression and psychosis. Illustrating the psychological roots to eating disorders, it places therapy within hospital, clinical and multi-disciplinary contexts, as well as displaying how psychoanalytic theory can be applied across various settings and in different teams.

Written by an eminent author in the field, this will be a key text for anyone wishing to understand eating disorders in children from a psychotherapeutic and psychoanalytic dimension.

Jeanne Magagna, PhD, is a child, adult and family psychotherapist trained at the Tavistock Clinic and former Head of Psychotherapy Services at Great Ormond Street Hospital. She currently teaches for the Centro Studi Martha Harris Tavistock Model trainings in Florence and Venice, Italy and is publishing and working internationally.

The Library of Child and Adolescent Psychoanalytic Psychotherapy
Series Editor: Jill Scharff

Recent titles in the series:

A Psychotherapeutic Understanding of Eating Disorders in Children and Young People: Ways to Release the Imprisoned Self
Jeanne Magagna

A Psychotherapeutic Understanding of Eating Disorders in Children and Young People

Ways to Release the Imprisoned Self

Jeanne Magagna

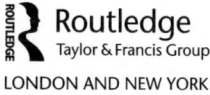

Routledge
Taylor & Francis Group

LONDON AND NEW YORK

First published 2022
by Routledge
2 Park Square, Milton Park, Abingdon, Oxon OX14 4RN

and by Routledge
605 Third Avenue, New York, NY 10158

Routledge is an imprint of the Taylor & Francis Group, an informa business

© 2022 Jeanne Magagna

British Library Cataloguing-in-Publication Data
A catalogue record for this book is available from the British Library

Library of Congress Cataloging-in-Publication Data
Names: Magagna, Jeanne, author.
Title: A psychotherapeutic understanding of eating disorders in children and young people : ways to release the imprisoned self / Jeanne Magagna.
Description: Milton Park, Abingdon, Oxon ; New York, NY : Routledge, 2022. | Series: The library of child and adolescent psychoanalytic psychotherapy | Includes bibliographical references and index. |
Identifiers: LCCN 2021019631 (print) | LCCN 2021019632 (ebook) | ISBN 9780367491901 (hardback) | ISBN 9780367491871 (paperback) | ISBN 9781003044970 (ebook)
Subjects: LCSH: Eating disorders in adolescence--Treatment. | Psychotherapy.
Classification: LCC RJ506.E18 M32 2022 (print) | LCC RJ506.E18 (ebook) | DDC 616.85/2600835--dc23
LC record available at https://lccn.loc.gov/2021019631
LC ebook record available at https://lccn.loc.gov/2021019632

ISBN: 978-0-367-49190-1 (hbk)
ISBN: 978-0-367-49187-1 (pbk)
ISBN: 978-1-003-04497-0 (ebk)

DOI: 10.4324/9781003044970

Typeset in Times New Roman
by Taylor & Francis Books

Contents

Figures

Foreword

I am delighted to feature this profound yet accessible book as the inaugural volume for the Library of Child Psychoanalytic Psychotherapy. I have seen Jeanne's skills in infant observation in a video teaching setting, where the learning group benefited from her empathy, attunement to affect and fantasy, and capacity for containment of the anxieties of those new to the study of early life. Jeanne proved to me that close observation of infant-parent interaction was not only fascinating, but essential for responding to primitive mental states affecting adult patients. Her co-authored books *Intimate Transformations: Babies with their Families* and *The Silent Child* carried forward that theme. Now comes *A Psychotherapeutic Understanding of Eating Disorders in Children and Young People.*

Jeanne Magagna comes to the writing of this volume from years of experience at intensive specialty units – from the giant paediatric hospital care at Great Ormond Street to the Tavistock Centre of excellence for child psychotherapy and infant observation. Jeanne is knowledgeable, empathic, persistent and optimistic. Her interventions are sensitive, compassionate, yet incisive. She fills her pages, and her treatments, with hope, born of experience and belief in the value of intensive psychoanalytic psychotherapy. She is a champion for growth of the imprisoned self.

Bringing a holistic psychoanalytic-systemic approach to understanding the interaction of mind, body, individual, peer group, and family in seriously ill children, she cares equally for those young people with impulses towards starvation, suicide and self-harm as for their parents without resorting to blame or giving in to despair. She does not shrink from hatred. Yet, she appeals to what is good and finds what is lively in each child and parent, and helps it grow. She cares as much for the verbal child who can speak her problems as for the silent, distrustful child who cannot or dare not find words for her distress. She knows how to reach behind the omnipotent grandiose self of the compulsive adolescent to the terrified infant protesting within the pubertal body. And she connects just as deeply with the helpless parents desperate for help. She shows that to do any effective work, she needs the cooperation of the parents in family meetings. These meetings may be dreaded at first but are soon found to be immensely useful.

Jeanne inspires us with her analytic sensibility, common sense and ability to resonate with the young person's vulnerability. She engages us with her terrific examples and powerfully evocative drawings to convey the child's distress and way of working through to health. She parses the elements of the complex presentation and aetiology of eating disorders and covers a range of conditions and ages: neurotic and psychotic; babies, latency age children and teenage girls and boys of various cultures. Some elements in the background coincide: many of the children have been found to be the result of an unplanned pregnancy and about a third of them reported having suffered sexual abuse. Various theories of unconscious motivation, conflict, and communication, including Klein, Bick, Bion, and Meltzer, are integrated into Jeanne's own approach. She draws on her countertransference to access the patient's and family's fear, hidden traumas, unexpressed rage, and frustrated desires, as shown in vivid illustrations of her work in process.

Having confronted the view that uncommunicative patients are unsuitable for talk therapy, Jeanne then proves to us that the work can be done. The way to do it is to work in a multidisciplinary team that offers attention to the social and family context, medical appraisal and monitoring of physical effects of severe mental illness, and individual listening, tuning in, and giving voice to the child's basic conflict particularly expressed in the transference. It is crucial to ask whether these silent children are hallucinating, and so get access to the voices of hidden persecutory parts of the self that drive the symptoms and thwart the treatment if they are not welcomed and harnessed to the task of recovery.

At all times, Jeanne is aware of the death anxiety that thins the air around treatment-refusing, underweight adolescents. She knows that they really can die, and that hospital care is essential as a physical support for psychological treatment. She describes marvellous individual psychoanalytic work, but she never overvalues it, always preferring to acknowledge the importance of the team approach. It takes a team to defeat the threat of death, support the life force and the expression of sexual desire and assertiveness, and free the imprisoned self.

It is time for this preface to let me go – I want to turn the page, and read this book again.

Jill Savege Scharff, M.D., Series Editor

Acknowledgements

I would like to thank Anne Alvarez and Donald Meltzer who have supervised much of this work and my psychoanalyst, Herbert Rosenfeld, who inspired me and supported me to do this very difficult task of being fully present with the young people and their families. Also, I very much appreciated Joshua Phillips who diligently helped me edit this book. I feel particularly grateful to Jill Savage Scharff, the editor of this series, for having invited me to make this contribution to the psychoanalytic study of eating disorders. My gratitude to Ellie Duncan and Alanna Donaldson for their very thoughtful editing of this book and to Susannah Frearson for overseeing this project.

I am also very grateful to the following for permission to publish these revised chapters:

Ch. 2. (2000), 'Severe eating difficulties: attacks on life', pp. 51–74. In: *Assessment in Child Psychotherapy*, Ed. Rustin, M. and Quagliata, E. London: Duckworth.

Ch. 3. (2007), 'Individual psychotherapy', pp. 257–295. In: Eds. Lask, B. and Bryant-Waugh, R. *Eating Disorders in Childhood and Adolescence* (2nd Edition). London: Routledge.

Ch. 3. Thank you also to Michael Leunig who speaks with pictures and has given permission to use his drawing, Figure 3.4, 'Listen to the heart'. Copyright Michael Leunig 1990.

Ch. 4. (1999), 'Il bambino interno e i genitori interni nella terapia familiare'. *Contrappunto*, 23: 3–21. Florence: Franco Cesati.

Ch 5. (1995), 'L'occhio rivolto all' interno', *Contrappunto*, 17: 61–82. Florence: Libreria Le Monnier.

Ch. 6. (2008), 'Attacks on life: suicidality and self-harm in young people'. In: Eds. Briggs, S., Lemma, A. and Crouch, W. *Relating to Self-Harm and Suicide*. London: Routledge.

Ch. 7. (2004), '"I didn't want to die but I had to": the pervasive refusal syndrome', pp. 107–139. In: Eds. Williams, G., Williams, H. and Desmarais Ravenscroft, K. *The Acceptance of Generosity: Eating Disorders in Children and Adolescents*. London: Karnac.

Ch. 8. (2018), 'The imprisoned self'. In *Counterdreamers: Analysts Reading Themselves.* Ed: Meg Harris Williams. London: The Harris Meltzer Trust.

Ch. 8. Thank you to Kathryn Harrison for permission to publish 'Mother's Day Card', found in (2003), *Seeking Rapture.* New York: Random House/ Routledge.

About the author

Jeanne Magagna was in the Eating Disorder Team and Head of Psychotherapy Services at Great Ormond Street Hospital of Children, London, for 24 years. While studying at the Tavistock Clinic in London she received three professional qualifications as a child, adult and family psychotherapist as well as obtaining a doctorate in psychotherapy in conjunction with the University of East London. She has held roles as vice-president and joint coordinator of the child psychotherapy Tavistock-Model trainings in the Centro Studi Martha Harris in Florence and Venice, Italy. Her edited books include: *Universals of Psychoanalysis* (1994), *The Silent Child: Communication without Words* (2012), *Creativity and Psychotic States* (2014), and her jointly edited books include: *Intimate Transformations: Babies with their Families* (2005), *Psychotherapy with Families* (1987), *Crises in Adolescence* (1994) and *Being Present for Your Nursery Age Child* (2014). She both publishes and teaches in person and through video links in many continents.

0000-0002-801506958

Introduction

From the time of conception onwards, the baby interacts with the emotional life of the mother, whose state of mind is affected by her relationship with her partner. In this intimate relationship with the mother, the body and psyche of the baby are transformed. Understanding derived from detailed observation of infants with their families forms the base of this book, designed to shed light on psychoanalytic work with children with eating difficulties and their families. There is a focus on the infantile experiences of the child in therapy and on how the infant-in-the-child is accepted, understood and transformed both through the relationship between the child and his/her parents in family therapy and the child and his individual psychotherapist. Described are therapeutic interactions between the therapist and eating disordered children and young people, which have at their base the emotional resonance stirred up in the psychotherapist's countertransference experiences with the child. The therapist's use of the countertransference, the main therapeutic method, involves receiving the child's experiences which may be present only in bodily states, actions or pictorial images and then enabling the child to find symbols and subsequently words suitable for meaningful and deep communication through words.

Described is the therapist's capacity for mentalization, which is similar to the tone of the mother's primary tasks, which is to use reverie to experience and then think about and meet the baby's physical and emotional needs, which include the baby's feeling of coldness, warmth, hunger, the need to be safely held and protected and the baby's need for intimacy with the parents. The collaborative attunement between mother and baby is the process through which the image of the body is constructed. The baby integrates perceptions and sensations of having physical and emotional needs met and forms an attachment to the caregiver. The chapters' many clinical vignettes portray how the therapist's understanding provides the eating disordered child with an opportunity to recover and develop infantile aspects of the psychological and physical self.

Most importantly, there is an emphasis on how the process of communication within the family and professional network surrounding the child requiring

DOI: 10.4324/9781003044970-1

therapy and in particular the external and internal family's way of supporting, containing and communicating emotional experiences create the foundation of this work. Perhaps what differentiates this book from other books on eating disorders is the focus on the child's relationships with the family from early infancy onwards. In particular, Chapter 1 (The theatre of the mouth) describes how the parents' relationship with their eating disordered child enables the child to mourn losses, work through conflictual issues or be a source of perpetual tension within the child because his or her feelings cannot be sufficiently elaborated upon and given emotional significance. The close similarities between the child's opening and closing of the mouth and the mind are shown through linking observations of four different babies with vignettes of children in psychotherapy. These examples include the collapsed crying mouth, the barricaded mouth, the gaping mouth and the terrified mouth. The focus is on the therapist's verbalized dialogue between his or her inner experience and the child's non-verbal bodily gestures and emotional states. Delineated also is the importance of the therapist allowing thoughts to be borne within herself through close observation, attunement and reverie rather than hanging onto already made thoughts from supervision, textbooks, and the first thought that forces itself, perhaps defensively, into one's mind.

In Chapter 2 (Ways of assessing children with severe eating difficulties), a six-year-old girl symbolizes the anxieties underlying her eating difficulties through drawing and talking about the scenes she has drawn. Early feelings about not tolerating the parental couple's togetherness as a source of anxiety are portrayed, as well as the primitive terrors of feeling insecurely held emotionally.

I feel that children suffering from a feeding or eating disorder deserve and their parents require some kind of psychotherapy – either parental work, family therapy or the child individually with ongoing parental work supporting the individual therapy (Magagna and Piercey, 2020). At one point, in the field of eating disorders, there existed a notion, which still exists in some places, that children should obtain good physical health before having therapy, have normal intelligence, show motivation to have therapy and be willing to speak. However, in the 2005 International Eating Disorder Conference in London, Tann (2005) described research on eating disordered patients facing compulsory admission and/or naso-gastric tube feeding. This research supports my long-held, but previously contentious belief, that whatever the motivation, the physical and mental condition of the severely eating disordered child, regardless of whether or not the child is speaking or motivated for change, he/she wants and deserves the opportunity to be spoken to and have his/her feelings respected and understood.

Because the anorectic symptoms of starving, non-stop exercise, feeling fat are so ubiquitous in anorexia nervosa, focusing solely upon these symptoms and using weight gain as a sign of health fails to address the severity of the psychopathology underneath anorexia nervosa. My 30 years of experience in eating disorders leads me to see that underneath the protective symptoms of anorexia nervosa there is a continuum of severity of anxieties ranging from psychotic to more neurotic and these anxieties need to be assessed alongside the eating disturbance symptomatology. Commonly found in the restricting anorectic children is an anxiety-ridden quest for perfection and obsessive compulsive symptomatology which pre-dated the onset of anorexia nervosa. Also, 75% of eating disordered people have an underlying depression (García-Villamisar et al., 2012).

As well as discussing less severe eating disturbances this book addresses that group of children for whom hospital admission is a necessity, both because of their life-risking physical condition and the inability of their families to assist them when they have such severe, often psychotic depression tinged with suicidal phantasies, as well as physically dangerous anorectic symptomatology. Outpatient services and private psychotherapists would generally not see these patients who arrive in the paediatric hospital because of the virtually continuous starvation and life-risking severe emaciation of the child's body, which is already lower than 65% weight-for-height or 14–15 BMI (body mass index). Although the clinical vignettes are mainly of girls, 27% of the children treated with severe eating disorders at Great Ormond Street Hospital have been boys.

In Chapter 3 (Individual psychotherapy in the context of a multidisciplinary eating disorder team) and the other psychotherapy-focused chapters, I describe how clinical work with eating disordered young people is facilitated by applying concepts derived from the close observation of infants in their families. It is through the study of infants that one can more profoundly understand the eating disordered child's primitive fears underlying their primitive protections which appear as anorectic symptoms. The children's primitive protections need to be relinquished in order to deepen their relationships with their external family members and subsequently internalize healthier adult figures to form a secure attachment to good, containing internal parental figures. Provided in the chapter is a view of the child's internal world and the way it changes as the child progresses in therapy. Illustrated is the child's developing capacity to depend upon and internalize the psychotherapist's and caregivers' capacity to bear and understand the child's feelings and primitive anxieties. At the time a child is particularly anxious in the therapy, the child repetitiously focuses on anorectic thoughts regarding calories, weight and shape. The therapist needs to find ways to avoid getting trapped into a monotonous dialogue about these topics by understanding the present moment in the therapy. In these chapters are three main contributions to the theory of my psychotherapy with eating disordered children: firstly, there is a description of the use of dreams as a means for clinicians to assess the child's psychic structure for bearing emotions; secondly, there is a description of the way in which through psychotherapy the child's hallucinations may be transformed from malevolent forces to benign processes, which can herald the possibility of internalization of a containing good figure; and thirdly, there follows a description of the parents' and eating disordered patient's total transference, which needs to be understood in the light of the psychotherapist's and multidisciplinary inpatient team's resulting countertransference responses.

Chapter 4 (Family therapy with a boy with eating disorders) demonstrates how parents and a therapist working within a multidisciplinary team can work as effective partners in helping the children who may communicate what needs to be understood, not verbally, but through projections into the family and staff and through psychosomatic activity such as vomiting, night-terrors and night-mares and anorexia nervosa. Family therapists often feel particularly troubled by what to do with the silent patient or younger child who cannot adequately describe sensations or emotions experienced both internally and within the family. One theme emphasized is that a child not speaking about his/her feelings need not prevent the child from feeling people are attempting to understand him/her. The use of structured spontaneity using play, drawings, dreams, stories and psycho-dramatic role playing is shown incorporated into my psychoanalytic family and individual psychotherapy. Alongside this is the acknowledgement of Mrs Bick's (1968) theory of observation of nonverbal communication. A focus in the therapist's sensitivity to the child and parents' most primitive anxieties and their need for protection in relation to them. Also shown is compassion for the ways in which the child and parents present themselves at each moment in the session.

Implicit throughout the book is my understanding that eating disorders are related to a profound disturbance in the child's early infantile life. My focus in the psychotherapy with eating disordered children is to work with their healthy inner resources to discover split-off parts of the body and emotional self and to work with the meaning of severe anxieties of either falling apart in a state of unintegration or disintegrating into a state of severe confusion. This falling apart and resort to eating difficulties is related to a disruption of containment in the relationship with the parental figures. Introjection of the parents' and psychotherapist's containing functions are described as the base for the child's therapeutic progress (Magagna and Piercey, 2020).

Theory surrounding eating disorders

The theoretical base of my psychotherapeutic work with people suffering from anorexia nervosa and/or a pervasive retreat from life is suffused pri-marily with the psychoanalytic ideas of Esther Bick, Melanie Klein, Wilfred Bion, Donald Meltzer and Herbert Rosenfeld. Susan Isaacs (1948) described how accompanying each bodily or emotional experience of the infant there is an unconscious phantasy which both influences how one relates to others and how one perceives the others relating to oneself. Both inside the womb and after birth, potentially the baby can have a sense of a benevolent space and later a good mother and father who provide physical holding, physical nurturance and emotional containment. Alongside this good experience are moments of experiencing a noxious space and later persecutory experiences linked with absence of a containing mother and father. The bad persecuting experiences are both in relation to the internalized parents and also in relation to mother's food into which the bad experiences get projected.

In normal development there is a predominance of good experiences over bad experiences, so that the mother is held in mind as a good mother who at times is frustrating and hated. The ambivalent relationship to the mother leads to both an emergence of concern for her and a wish to protect her or repair the phantasied damage done to her. Through the repeated experience of having the mother or primary caregiver empathically receive the baby's intense emotional experiences, hold them in mind, and through a process of her reverie giving meaning to them, the baby internalizes a 'holding mother'. This internalization of a holding, containing mother becomes the base for the creation of an internal space comprised of internal objects to whom one relates. Throughout life, the child's relationship to internal mother, father, siblings then informs each interactions with his family and the outside world. Described in these chapters are the internal and external relationships of eating disordered children between the ages of six to 18.

Pervasive retreat from life

Children pervasively retreating from life regress to not eating, not walking, not talking, not moving and both physically and psychologically not opening their eyes to the outside world. In Chapter 5 (The eye turned inward) one child, as she was recovering, described the experience of pervasive retreat through a dream. The dream depicted her brain being removed and placed 'in a vase'. This suggests that in the case of someone pervasively retreating, the whole of the self is encapsulated in a claustrum of 'not thinking' while regression reaches back to the foetal position of entering and residing 'inside the object' or inside the mother (Meltzer, 1992). Some of the illest of the 17 pervasively retreating children whom I have seen for family and/or individual psychotherapy have regressed to a situation in which there is no memory of words or numbers, no memory of the past or recollection of the family home or family members. The child's regression is back to a complete 'not knowing', an obliteration of the external world.

The pervasive retreat presents an extreme version of the child's withdrawal from the intimacy of human relationships and food and drink necessary for life itself. Withdrawal into a 'claustrum' away from any experience of the stimuli of food or human contact can be seen as a life-protective mechanism saving the self from further encounters with adverse inner or outer emotional experiences. This dissociation (Krystal, 1978) and (Meltzer, 1992) follows when there is a failure of 'second skin phenomena' (Bick, 1968) to 'hold the unintegrated parts of the self together' in order to survive the 'nameless dread' of death and disintegration and psychosis.

Meltzer (1992), Garber and Seligman (1980), Nunn and Thompson (1996) and Nunn et al. (2014) have all informed my work with these pervasively retreating children. At times I was left wondering if the children's numbing of responsiveness, reduced involvement with the external world, pervasively diminished interest in the normal activities of daily life and severely constricted emotions was linked with a pervasive sense of helplessness as part of a post-traumatic stress disorder (Garber and Seligman, 1980). At other times, I sensed that separation anxiety (Nunn and Thompson, 1996) was a prominent feature accompanied by social withdrawal, depression and a hopelessness that it would be possible to influence difficult situations relating to the health, safety and happiness within the family. Meltzer describes how the delusional world of living 'in the claustrum', as pervasively retreating children do, involves failed containment, lack of symbol formation and a dread of mental life: 'parts of the personality come to live in this "nowhere" world of the delusional system' (Meltzer, 1992, p. 118).

These silent, unmoving pervasively retreating children with little adequate mental functioning, throughout the course of hospitalisation lasting a year to 18 months, oscillate between peeking out towards life and relationships with significant others and a move backwards to being in a foetal position, inside the object, seemingly unaware of the self and others. Gradually the children find their way back into using adhesive mechanisms and with the help of family and individual psychotherapy are generally able to resume relationships with school, friends and family. This is described in Chapter 7 (Pervasive retreat). The basic therapeutic method involves being attuned to the emotional experience of being with the non-speaking child both in the session and in the therapeutic milieu to make sense of the child's experience. The therapeutic team and parents need to work together to make sense of the child's projections of physical and emotional states. Applying Bick's (1968) observational approach of empathic attentiveness to minute aspects of the child's nonverbal dialogue with the therapist involves right brain to right brain therapeutic communication, considered by Schore (2002) to be the first point of therapeutic action.

The consideration and later verbalization of my countertransference responses to the child's primitive experiences, including sensations and movement or stillness of her body, was essential for the child, before he/she could put these experiences into a symbolic form for communication (Magagna, 2012). Empathic understanding of the child permits an integration of the child's body and psychological self. Internalization of the therapist's state of mind enabled each of these 17 children to begin a process of mentalization. As the children gradually made their exit from 'the claustrum', the residence involving massive projection of self into the object, they resorted to adhesive mechanisms and appeared in some ways similar to children suffering from anorexia nervosa. There is an attentive self emerging and depending on the thinking functions of the caregiver, nurse and therapist. However, if the emotional experience is too intense, too conflictual, too different to be contemplated, there is a return to adhesive clinging to save the self from disintegration and terror (Emanuel, 2001).

Aetiology and inner structures underlying severe, restricting eating disorders

External, physiological and genetic factors

According to a 2019 British Medical Journal publication of research done in 2015, anorexia nervosa is prevalent in about 5% of females, with a mean age of 14.6. The incidence of anorexic young people under 12 is increasing. About 9% of the young eating disordered people are boys and 92% are white (Petkova et al., 2019). Anorexia nervosa is rare in underdeveloped countries, often appearing for the first time during rapid social change in different cultures (ibid., p. 177). In this research, anorexia nervosa is defined as the pursuit of thinness through dietary restriction and other weight-control measures resulting in a BMI of 15, substantially below the normal range which is around 20 BMI. Anorexia nervosa is 'organized around a characteristic set of beliefs about the importance of weight as an index of perceived worth' (ibid., p. 177).

As well as the predisposing factors, including possible genetic factors (Treasure and Holland, 1989) and a faulty inner psychic structure, there may be a 'triggering' event, possibly related to the physiological changes associated with puberty. Among these physiological body changes is the fact that brain development of intellectual functions occurs more slowly than the surge of feelings in puberty (Nelson et al., 2005, p. 70). Also, various other factors, such as physical abuse, emotional abuse and sexual abuse, may cause the breakdown of an already faulty psychic structure which has been prompting general dissatisfaction with life and the self. Approximately 30–40% of the anorectic young people coming to our eating disorders team have been sexually abused. The presence of a harsh superego coupled with the fact that, prior to participating in psychotherapy, very few of them have been able to trust anyone sufficiently to tell them about the abuse, may contribute to their distress surrounding the abuse. There may also be bullying, the infliction of a narcissistic wound, and extreme anxieties associated with perfectionism and competition at school. Also loss of father's employment and marital distress of the parents are contributory factors (Wren and Lask, 1993). Being projected into with negative emotions by family members or others can also be a factor contributing to the formation of a young person's anorectic symptomatology.

Internal psychological structures

Underlying similar anorectic symptoms of starving and severe weight loss are different psychological protections, which vary from moment to moment according to the severity of the child's anxieties and the child's capacity to bear their intensity and conflictual nature. In the various chapters there are descriptions of the following protections and defences: (a) living in the claustrum, (b) double identifications, (c) adhesive clinging, and (d) obsessive omnipotent control.

Living in the claustrum

Children suffering from pervasive retreat and the severest types of anorexia nervosa first reside 'inside the object', with a delusional psychic structure that involves massive projective identification into the object. Emanuel (2001, p. 1069) describes 'the potentially annihilating terror implicit in the experience of contact with the void – the domain of the non-existent or nothingness, conceived as immensely hostile object, terrifying space or a place of "nameless dread"'. Petrelli (2003) also describes an anorectic girl's paralysing sense of emptiness. All manifestations of existence are threatened by contact with the void, necessitating the deployment of a variety of defences. These defences include trying to search for a fixed sense of identity, which can often propel people to seek refuge inside an object or state of mind, as described by Meltzer's (1992) 'claustrum' and by Steiner's 'psychic retreat'.

It is clear from many young people's descriptions that the entry into anorectic delusional thinking and activity is designed to save the self from fragmentation, loss of the self through psychotic confusional states and anxieties. (Fenichel, 1945)

Adhesive identification

Esther Bick (1968) describes the terrifying fear of annihilation, disintegration and falling which in the absence of the 'holding mother' prompt the infant to cling adhesively to the surface of objects, parts of the body, a noise, become rigid, motionless, or get involved in non-stop leg and arm movements to 'hold the self together', forming 'a second skin'.

Repeated turning to adhesive mechanisms which involve 'depending on the self' rather than on the containing functions of the mother leads to a very primitive infantile self being held in an encapsulated, split-off form. This occurs in extremely difficult situations, linked with the infant's phantasies and/or the actual detrimental lack of an emotionally containing relationship provided by the primary caregiver. For example, as shown in Chapter 1, a young infant hit by her brother may become rigid, motionless, stare blankly, dissociate from the external experience as a way of surviving the traumatic relationship. Repeated trauma can lead to a more frequent return to 'not thinking' as a method of surviving adversity. This also occurs in extremely difficult situations, linked with the infant's phantasies and/or the actual detrimental lack of containment provided by the primary caregiver. This often occurs when incubated premature infants are not looked after adequately.

It is vital to recognize the inner state of eating disordered young people and in particular the presence of their powerful psychotic anxieties (Farrell, 1995). A move from fear of breakdown to holding onto omnipotent control of starving, non-stop exercising, shutting the door to others' emotions and those of the self (Emanuel, 2001) is initially experienced as a relief from intense suffering.

Double identification

The massive projection of the self into the maternal object involves a double identification (Rey, 1994). Firstly, the self intrudes into and identifies with the body of an attacked and damaged mother. Secondly, there is an identification with the baby self, which resides inside the mother and is bulging with the young person's intense, uncontained emotions. This phenomenon contributes to the bodily experience of being fat and ugly and experiencing low self-esteem. Such feelings are extremely common in the anorectic children aged six to 18 seen in individual, family and group therapy. Starvation seems to be a method of trying to deny and control the bad internal mother. There is a fear of growing bigger, fatter, more greedy.

In other situations, a baby or older child who is unable to bear the frustration of not having her needs or wishes met by the mother may feel rage and anger towards the mother. As a result of the infant's sadism the mother is experienced as being filled with projections of bad feelings and hence experienced as bad. The bad mother becomes a persecutory figure and both the bad mother and the food representing her are rejected. This contributes to the child's difficulty with eating.

Obsessive omnipotent control

Palazzoli (1978) suggests that starvation can sometimes be used as an attempt to deny and achieve control over 'the bad mother' through being autonomous. However, her idea of the young person striving for autonomy overlooks the idea that the anorectic young person is really using primitive omnipotence because she has not introjected the mentalizing functions of the parental figures that would enable her to achieve mature autonomy rather than pseudo-autonomy.

In early infancy, as described by Bick (1968), but also in later development, including puberty, there is a use of omnipotent control which somewhat later becomes obsessive. At the time of puberty, when typically anorexia nervosa is more frequent, one's brain structure changes (Nelson et al., 2005, p. 170) with a mismatch between the maturation of the affective node of the brain and the cognitive-regulatory node, which lags behind by several years. As the brain and body are changing, the actual physical structure of the latency age body may be held onto for security in an adhesive or controlling way. The child can feel there are just too many changes in the body and menstruation can be experienced as the spontaneously maturing body's attack on the child's need for control. As a result, the child may start starving after the first menstruation.

In puberty, not only do the body structure and physiological responses change, but there are also developmental changes fostering independence from the family and closer ties with the peer group. These major life changes pose a challenge to the pre-existing fragile internalized capacities of young people as they form attachments to their peer group and spend more time away from the family. As a result, an experience of identification with a damaged maternal body psychotic thinking and/or anorexia nervosa can occur (Laufer, 1981, p. 68).

One of Dr Henri Rey's patients put the problem of resorting to obsessive, omnipotent control succinctly, saying:

> Although I denied it initially, I have had to accept the painful truth that the changes of puberty, the increase in size, shape and eight, menstruation and new and disturbing impulses, all presented a dangerous challenge for which I was unprepared and which threatened what little control I had. To counteract this fear of losing control, I resorted to rigid dieting and became preoccupied with weight.
>
> (Rey, 1994, p. 63)

Behind the omnipotent control there is a move to a position of denial of psychic pain, absence of thinking (Bion, 1962) and encapsulation. The anorectic young person uses omnipotent control rather than mentalization (Fonagy et al., 2004). Using omnipotent control means that alongside the rejection of food is withdrawal from intimacy with both one's infantile emotional life and intimate encounters with primary family figures including mother, father and siblings upon whom one depends. Also, therapy, which like food is a required part of treatment for recovery, is generally perceived as a threat to the omnipotent structure controlling food intake as well as the expression of emotions.

The 'encapsulated self' (S. Klein, 1980) that is overusing primitive protections against anxiety has been depicted in one anorectic girl's drawings as a bear, with a noose around his neck, locked in a prison. Another girl drew herself in a prison cell, crying, with her back turned to her mother who was standing outside the cell but was locked out and could not enter the cell to help her child.

The fear of fatness

As a result of an experience of identification with a damaged maternal body psychotic thinking and/or anorexia nervosa can occur. Orbach (1994) states that the anorectic young person feels her body is not right. She goes on to say that mismatching in the relationship between mother and daughter, and also between mother and son, provides the precondition for symptomatology that includes body-image distortion. The attempt to 'make the body thin' is an attempt to repair this damaged self identified with the deformed, bulging damaged maternal object. The wish is for a thin, beautiful body separate from and in introjective identification with a well-formed, beautiful mother/woman. This drive is not only for thinness and beauty, for there is also a wish for happiness. 'When I am thin, then I will be happy' is often stated by anorectic girls in the initial assessment. A child's drawing showing this experience of 'fatness' is to be found in Chapter 3, discussing individual psychotherapy. In both anorectic boys and girls the enlargement of the body-self and the feelings of fatness are caused by overwhelming, uncontained feelings of depression, rage and/or a sense of loneliness (Magagna, 1994). Ways of considering and containing those painful feelings are depicted in Magagna (2004).

One young person said:

> When I eventually weighed under 80 pounds [about 36 kilos] and looked at myself in the mirror ... I saw someone beautiful. I saw myself. ... The clearer the outline of my skeleton became, the more I felt my true self to be emerging ... I was, literally and metaphorically, in perfect shape ... I was so superior that I considered myself to be virtually beyond criticism.
>
> (Macleod, 1982, pp. 68–79)

Clearly, the anorectic person had become attached to the bones of the anorectic self as 'the true and best self' (Vitousek, 2005), and yet this 'true self' is involved in the attachment to a 'false self' of primitive protections against anxiety. The attempt to 'make the body thin' is an attempt to repair this damaged self, identified with the deformed, bulging, damaged maternal object. The wish is for a thin, beautiful body separate from, but experienced in introjective identification with a well-formed, beautiful mother/woman.

In the case of a boy, such as the boy described in Chapter 4, there is also a sense of fatness. In the boys who comprised 27% of treatment population Great Ormond Street Hospital treatment population, they said they wished to get rid of the 'flab' and hold onto 'hard muscle and bone'. I sense that the flab, representing damaged internalized parents, does not feel connected to any bone structure representing inner psychic structures. Instead the 'flab' seems to represent unformed, unstructured 'stuff' of undigested emotions which overwhelm the psyche. A male anorectic described his rationale for dieting, saying:

> I hated my physical appearance because, no matter what I did, I was still fat and ugly. I was drowning in self-disgust ... I was deeply depressed ... I was completely imprisoned by anorexia. It isolated me but it allowed me to operate in a world that was totally counter to the dialogue of worthlessness in my head ...
>
> (Eccleston, 2019, pp. 114–116)

In both the anorectic boys and girls whom I have seen, 'the unstructured stuff', the sense of fatness, includes a predominance of uncontained intense rage, depression, a sense of inner damage and loneliness. Orbach confirms what I have stated, saying, 'The anorectic girl's hatred of her body is a reflection of a more general kind of self hate, despair and hopelessness not able to be experienced directly' (1994, p. 173). She says this hatred of the body needs to be accepted, and thus authenticated, 'not by accepting the patient's definition of the body, but by receiving the patient's experience of it ... there is no use persuading the young girl that her experience is different than it is' (ibid., p. 174). In this way the young person will begin to integrate a psychosomatic sense of the self. For this reason it seems therapeutically helpful to start from where the young person is and accept the experience of the body as being ugly, hated and the potential source of happiness if transformed. The therapist's further exploration of the distress regarding the body can lead to more generalisation of what feels so distressing.

Striving for happiness

The anorectic young person's drive is not only for thinness and beauty; there is also a wish for happiness. 'When I am thin, then I will be happy' is often stated by the anorectic young people during their initial assessment phase. Understanding the young person's goals and wishes for happiness beyond the wish for 'thinness' and lending a hand towards thinking about ways of reaching these goals is part of the motivational aspects of therapy which Geller (Geller et al., 2001) has found to be so successful in treating people with chronic anorectic behaviour.

My approach to working with eating disordered young people: liaison between professionals

In working psychoanalytically with eating disordered young people I place an emphasis on a systemic view of the interrelationship between the capacity for nurturing, protecting and mentalizing of the present in the parents, the multidisciplinary team, including the individual psychotherapist, and the anorectic child's inner world (Box et al., 1981). I advocate the inclusion of the simultaneous occurrence of family and individual psychotherapy and parents' groups when possible. I also suggest following the NICE 2018 guidelines, which recommend that medical and diet issues as well as weight monitoring take place in the same location or with regular liaison between nurse/doctor and the family therapist. This involves having a doctor or nurse directly involved in taking the child's pulse, checking physical extremities and discussing other medical issues with the child and family.

For example, I recommend that another team member weigh the child and report directly to the family therapists, who can chart and discuss weight changes with the young person and parents in connection with other developments in the therapies. The function of her anorectic symptoms is looked at moment to moment in her discussions with the therapist, for discussion of weight often unconsciously occurs to evade emotional experiences in relation to a topic which being considered (Chapter 3).

Analysis of the patient's transfer of internalized significant people onto the therapist and the countertransference phenomena includes discussing weight loss and weight gain as part of the transference to the therapist (Dare and Crowther, 1995). For example, frequently weight loss occurs when the child feels the loss of the therapist during holidays.

Working with the unconscious

Psychoanalytic therapy involves working with unconscious elements in the child's personality. My psychotherapeutic approach with severely eating disordered children has been influenced by psychoanalytic ideas of Bick (1962, 1964, 1968), Bion (1962), Meltzer (1967, 1992) and Schore (2002). Also, I am particularly grateful to Anne Alvarez, specially known for her work in autism and borderline states, whose theories and supervisions have informed my work with eating disordered children.

Susan Isaacs (1948) described how accompanying each of the infant's bodily or emotional experience there is an unconscious phantasy. Unconscious phantasy influences how one relates to others and also how one perceives others relating to oneself. Both inside the womb and after birth, the baby potentially can have a sense of a benevolent space and later, a good mother who provides physical holding, physical nurturance and emotional containment. Alongside this good experience are moments when the infant experiences noxious experiences, which get projected and are followed by persecutory anxieties. Also, the infant experiences deep fears of annihilation and persecution in the absence of a containing mother.

In normal development there is a predominance of good experiences over bad experiences so that the mother is held in mind as a good mother who at times is frustrating and hated. The child's ambivalent relationship to the mother leads to an emergence of both concern for her and a wish to protect her or repair the phantasied damage done to her. Through the repeated experience of having the mother or primary caregiver empathically receive the baby's intense emotional experiences, hold them in mind and through the process of her reverie, giving meaning to them, the baby internalizes a 'holding mother'. This internalization of a holding, containing mother becomes the base for the creation of an internal space comprised of 'internal parents' (called 'objects' in psychoanalysis) to whom one relates. Throughout life, the person's relationship to the internal mother, father and siblings then informs each interaction with her family and the outside world (Cooper and Magagna, 2005).

Any person suffering from an eating disorder does not simply turn away from food. Alongside the rejection of food is withdrawal from intimacy and thoughtfulness in relation to one's infantile emotional life. I have seen a large number of eating disordered young people and been part of many discussions in Gianna Williams' Tavistock Clinic Eating Disorder Workshop, which published two volumes entitled *The Generosity of Acceptance* (Williams et al., 2004), to which I contributed.

Dubinsky (2004) describes the main theoretical understanding contained in *The Generosity of Acceptance* when speaking of an anorectic girl who

> did not have an internal or external mother who was in touch with the child's needs, who could process anxieties, help her to understand them and enable her to feel nurtured and contained. Her internal mother did not seem able to tolerate the needs of a hungry, demanding chid with needs of her own. Rather, she perceived the chid not only as an extension of herself in which she *can* project her own needs, anxiety and persecution, but also as a threatening rival ... in adolescence (the young person) started to say 'no' to food ... 'no' to the fear of her mother's unpredictable moods and projections ... When she turned her back on food, she turned away from that which is life-sustaining; omnipotent control over herself and her objects took its place ... She saw it as a means of exerting obsessional control over her needs, which threatened to overwhelm her.
>
> (pp. 190–191)

Focus on the transference and countertransference

Most obvious in the chapters is a description of both the psychotherapist's countertransference as a therapeutic instrument and the psychotherapist's and team's own difficulties which might impact on the child. I am interested in the containing function which the psychotherapist offers to the young person at each particular moment in the therapy and what the young person makes of what is offered by the psychotherapist. I am asking myself, 'Does the young person evade what is being discussed, evacuate and project feelings arising or manage to take in the therapist's interpretations?' I use my counter-transference experiences to understand these reciprocal interactions. Whether the child is responding with a defensive rejection of what is offered because the therapist has mis-attuned by going too deep and or touching something too painful to bear or whether the child responds with a grateful acceptance of what is offered by the therapist requires exploration of the ongoing dynamics between the child and the psychotherapist.

Particularly in inpatient psychotherapy work it is essential to take note of using the total transference, described in Chapter 3. As the children suffering from pervasive refusal and anorexia nervosa gradually exit from the delusional structure of their illness involving massive projective identification into the object, they resort to adhesive mechanisms. There is an attentive self emerging with dependence on the therapist's and nurses' benevolent empathic thinking functions. However, if the emotional experience is too intense, too conflictual, too different to be contemplated, there is a return to pervasive withdrawal, adhesively clinging to retreat or obsessive anorectic symptomatology.

Understanding the total transference to the institution and providing group discussions in daily community meetings in which each person is expected to speak and be heard three or four times helps promote the idea that the whole community including all staff is thinking about the emotional needs of each child and this communal activity reduces acting out. Family and individual therapy which also addresses the important aspects of the sibling relationship, including helpful and damaging aspects of the sibling friendship and competitive jealousy, can also promote health rather than regression to illness. Similarly, if the family reduces their high expressed emotions there is less chance for regression when the child relates to their family. Family members with high expressed emotion are hostile, very critical and not tolerant of their anorectic child's behaviour. They feel like they are helping by having this attitude. They not only criticize behaviours relating to the eating disorder but also other behaviours that are unique to the personality of the child. High expressed emotion is more likely to cause a relapse than low expressed emotion. The three dimensions of high expressed emotion are hostility, emotional over-involvement and critical comments (Vaughn and Leff, 1985).

The fear of turning to the mother and her food is that the mother will be unreliable, unavailable, frustrating, not able or willing to meet the needs of the developing infantile self. The young person's lacking a good internal container for holding feelings leads to enslavement to overwhelming feelings including anger, sadness, and an intense longing to be understood and loved completely by the primary caregiver. Although competitiveness with the mother and/or father and envy of the mother (Sohn, 1985, p. 51) might form part of the damage to the internalized mother, it is also very important to consider that attacking the mother's babies, one's siblings, leading to damaged internal siblings, damaged mother and possessiveness of the mother. This competitive relationship to siblings as well as the parents, accompanied by attacks on the frustrating mother and father, are a prominent and sometimes neglected feature in young people suffering from anorexia nervosa (Wright, 2004 and Magagna, 2005).

As physical health is restored and psychological progress occurs, the experience of residing in an inpatient unit with eight to 20 inpatients can influence the emergence of infantile transferences from the family: increased competitiveness through use of the symptoms of the illness can present a real threat to the young person's progress. For example, a young person may begin eating fairly normally, make psychological progress facilitating discharge, but then her psychotherapist or keyworker nurse is assigned to a new emaciated, self-harming, anorectic patient. This can foster a notion that the therapeutic workers are going to be too involved with the iller child, representing mother's new baby, and find themselves unavailable to her. Such possessive jealousy can prompt attacks on the body through cutting, starving, return to pervasive retreat and anorectic symptomatology of the past. Aspects of the move from anorexia nervosa to other methods of self-harm are shown in Chapter 6 (Suicidal and self-harm ideation accompanying eating disorders). Through this regression the young person attempts to compete with the illest child through making an impact by creating anxiety in the staff who have turned bad through jealousy. It is at this point that the anorectic child might say, 'You aren't hearing me' or 'You don't really care, it's only a job' or 'You only pay attention to the iller child'.

Factors impeding the anorectic child's progress in psychotherapy

Attachment to the false self

As the young person is developing some insight in psychotherapy, it feels like two pathways are available. Firstly, there is the path of 'attachment to the false self' (Magagna and Segal, 1990) involving the anorectic child's addiction to omnipotent protective measure that include control of food intake and/or an 'internal gang' (Rosenfeld, 1971 and Meltzer, 1973) attacking the goodness of the inner object and the good external figures upon whom the child relies. At this point 'I just want to die' is frequently stated by some anorectic young people. Death is presented by 'the internal gang' as a solution to the misery of life. However, anorectic young people who, without the intervention of their parents and/or professionals might starve to death, seem to hear but not believe that starvation brings death and the complete annihilation of the self.

For example, one eating disordered adolescent wanted to die in order to be in non-stop conversation with her God in heaven (Magagna, 1988). Another girl, a twin, wanted to die because she experienced no emotional point to her existence on earth and felt that through dying she would enter a state of comforting plea-sure. Also, even when wasting, at 57% weight-for-height, an anorectic girl maintained the phantasy that with her mind she could transcend her body (Palazzoli, 1978). Primitive omnipotence can lead to a belief that the self is beyond normal human predicaments associated with life and death.

Secondly, there is the more frightening, painful process of risking dependency on intimate, thoughtful encounters with the therapist, parents and the mother's food which is a concrete representation of nurturance to the dependent baby self. This process is shown in Chapter 3 regarding developments in individual psychotherapy.

It is important for a psychotherapist thinking about the young person's reluctance to come to therapy to remember that the therapeutic relationship may involve transference of the young person's fear of turning to her actual or internalized mother and her food. The fear is that the mother will be unreli-able, unavailable, frustrating, not able or willing to meet the needs of the developing infantile self. The young person, lacking a good internal container for holding feelings, fears enslavement to overwhelming feelings, including anger, sadness and an intense longing to be understood and loved completely by the primary caregiver. These feelings can get transferred onto the therapist as the therapeutic relationship develops.

Presence of a harsh superego

What is striking is that the destructive aims towards mother, father and siblings are most frequently unconscious or at least hidden in overt interactions with the family. The repression of one's destructiveness into the unconscious is dictated by the harsh superego which blames the self for having negative feelings towards others. This promotes persecutory guilt, making the anorectic young person feel a bad person, not deserving of anything good, including food, presents and parental love. However, there is also a splitting-off of the destructive self and projection of aggression onto others and also onto food, a symbol of mother's nurturance. When denial of aggression and other conflictual feelings toward external figures occur, there is an accompanying damage to the internal objects creating persecutory anxieties. This has usually been a part of personality development prior to the onset of either pervasive retreat or anorexia nervosa. Nightmares, sleeplessness linked with persecutory dreams filled with damaged internal objects usually surround anorexia nervosa (Magagna and Segal, 1990).

Addiction to sadomasochism

Anorectic young people are often addicted to sadomasochistic encounters with others or with their cruel superego. 'This cruelty to the self and one's objects is often used as an antidote to despair ... the excitement engendered by it can feel like imbuing greyness with colour albeit of a disturbing nature' (Emanuel, 2001). Such a relationship with a cruel sadistic superego leaves one devoid of the pleasure of spontaneous play, work or relationships with others.

Subsequently there occurs an external event, or the physiological changes associated with puberty, including brain intellectual functioning developing more slowly than the surge of feelings in puberty. The external events may include sexual abuse, as has been the case with 30–40% of the anorectic population, bullying, someone causing a narcissistic wound causing the breakdown of an already faulty psychic structure. Attaching oneself to the cruel voice of the perfectionist self as one pursues one's academic pursuits in a competitive way with others can also be a form of sadomasochism. One is constantly berated for not being perfect and constantly trying to top other high achieving students' performance.

Competition with 'the third person' and, ultimately, an attack on the parental couple

We have described the influence of competition with the third person, whether it be sibling or father or mother in Magagna and Owen (2011). Feeling very possessive of mother contributes to attacking the 'mother's babies, one's siblings, resulting in damaged internal siblings and thus a damaged mother'

(Cooper and Magagna, 2005). 'Ganging up' with a sibling occurs to avoid both the frustrations of possessiveness and dependence on the mother or the father and competitive oedipal rivalry.

Sohn (1985, p. 51) describes how envy or possessiveness towards one or both of the parents may prompt an accompanying attack on the parental couple. Such an attack is also described in Lawrence's paper 'Loving them to death: The anorectic and her objects', where she states: 'Whenever one meets a patient in the grip of anorexia nervosa, one knows that some kind of cata-strophe has taken place' (2001, p. 44). She explains how the internal objects have been internalized but attacked in such a way that they are permanently in thrall, suspended or frozen. Lawrence is positing a method of obsessive control of and attack upon the internalized couple while indicating that there is a need 'to buttress manic defences against depressive pain associated with the reality of the oedipal situation' (ibid., p. 44).

Parents intrusively entering with projections of their mental states

Also in Lawrence's work (2001) there is a countertransference experience of the patient's emptiness and inner deadness. This is in contrast to that evocation of a wish to be helped described by Gianna Williams in her paper on 'no-entry defences' (1997, p. 78). In that paper, Williams goes beyond Dubinsky's (2004) notion of the lack of a good containing internal mother, for she describes how an anorectic child may feel not only uncontained but also perceive herself as a receptacle of the parents' projections of unmetabolized phantasies and experi-ences. Likierman (1997) also describes a mutually destructive link between mother and child when the mother is unable to meet the child's needs. Williams and Likierman indicate this can contribute to the child dreading dependence on the mother. Williams et al. (2004) go on to suggest that if the child is open to her parents' projections, she may internalize an agent which performs a dis-organising disrupting function, which is the opposite function to emotionally containing experiences. Williams also indicates that these children will convey a wish to be helped to clean up some mess and to find a thinking, organizing mental function.

Recovery from anorexia

'Will there ever be a recovery from anorexia nervosa or symptoms of pervasive retreat?' In the *Oxford Textbook of Psychotherapy*, Vitousek and Gray (2005) indicate that anorectic individuals are much less likely to seek treatment, to persevere in efforts to change and to obtain benefit even if they remain engaged. My 30 years of experience providing family, individual and group therapy for children and their parents is very different. Only a few of the young people leave psychotherapy prematurely and few do not recover from anorexia nervosa if they are willing to participate in psychoanalytic psychotherapy long enough.

Generally the required psychotherapeutic individual and family work is from 18 months to two and a half years. Most of the eating disorder literature on therapeutic success assumes that the young person will have become a normal weight-for-height percentile, stopped vomiting, purging, excessive exercising and starving, let go of the obsessional need for control and achieved a healthy sense of self-identity which is not based on anorexia and thinness. In the psychoanalytic literature, Quagliata (2002) and Williams et al. (2004) assume that in addition to these external criteria for recovery, the harsh, cruel superego would be modified and the overuse of adhesive protections, particularly omnipotent control, would be replaced by the stabilizing presence of an improved psychic structure consisting of good internal parental figures. These identifications with good internal parental figures would provide a solid inner core from which would emanate good self-esteem, in identification with these good internalized parents, and the capacity to bear mental pain.

Chapter 3, which describes developments in individual psychotherapy, suggests that a young person is required to forgive the parents, take responsibility for thinking about her own loving and destructive feelings towards internal and external family members, and make efforts towards repairing relationships. Externally visible should be the diminution of severe weight and shape concerns, perfectionism, low self-esteem, mood intolerance and interpersonal difficulties. At times during psychotherapy, and sometimes following it, there may be circumstances that make it appropriate for the young person to live separately from the family for short or lengthier periods of time. Adverse factors in the family which are felt to be emotionally or physically abusive may lead the anorectic young person, and perhaps other members for the family, to develop a 'no-entry' system of defences (Williams, 1997) which ultimately impedes emotional development.

The anorectic young person in family therapy

Parents of anorectic young people inevitably feel they are to blame for not providing 'good enough parenting' to meet their child's emotional needs. Professionals note the failures in providing effective parenting, but they are often seeing a family who has become dysfunctional during many weeks or months of their anorectic child being ill. Regardless of the situation it is obvious that blaming either the child or the parents or their anorectic child promotes further family dysfunction (Lask and Bryant-Waugh, 1993). It is useful to approach the child's anorexia with an attitude of being curious and trying to understand ways of ameliorating the difficulties in the family.

My own therapeutic approach to families and their anorectic child is to consider a systemic view in which there is an examination of the interrelationship between the primary caregivers and the child's inner world and constitutional characteristics (Box et al., 1994). Mentalization (Bateman and Fonagy, 2004) of affective states and their modulation through reverie are essential for emotional growth of a healthy personality. The psychotherapist's task is to recover the family's capacity for mentalization and heal the mismatch of communication between the family and the anorectic young person as shown in Chapter 4. In this chapter I gain access to the unconscious mental life of the silent anorectic child's family through play, drawings, dreams and psychodrama techniques.

The clinical example presented contradicts existing famiy therapy notions of 'the anorectic young person's quest for autonomy' (Palazzoli, 1974). The chapter shows how destructive pseudo-autonomy, masked as 'hard work', is used as a defence against the experiences of love, loss, hurt and hate. The family's pseudo-autonomy (Bick, 1968), as part of the psychic structure using adhesive mechanisms, lends importance to looking into the unconscious experiences and psychological development underlying the family's apparently normal surface behaviours including the child's resumption of eating. This is accomplished through observation of both the family's nonverbal and verbal communication and acute sensitivity, through use of the countertransference, to each child's and parent's most primitive anxieties, present from moment to moment in the session.

My model of family therapy is enriched by the re-establishment or strengthening of parental authority, helping the parents work cooperatively with the child, restructuring family relationships so that conflicts other than the eating disorder dominate the picture and helping the child to maintain a healthy weight. This method of working is in some ways similar to family therapy proposed by Dare and Eisler (1995); however, it is a new contribution to family therapy because it specifically focuses on the inner world while incorporating creative psychoanalytic techniques for working with the younger, silent young person and/or younger siblings. Often attention is paid to the family and child's developmental phase and to role conflicts and changes as well as the family's capacity for mentalization, which may have been impeded for generations. Empathic understanding must be given to the parents, who may themselves be attempting to ward off psychic pain regarding their own relationship and lost and disturbed relationships with their own parents (Bozszormenyi-Nagy Spark, 1973; Schutzenberger, 1998).

The family system may be such that emotions are emitted, projected with few emotional experiences being contained (Zinner and Shapiro, 1972). In this situation, the anorectic young person and perhaps other members of the family may develop a 'no-entry' system of defences (Williams, 1997). The therapist showing compassionate understanding of the family's primitive protections in relation to anxiety fosters a modulation of the ferocity of the critical superego functioning within the family system.

Alongside family therapy it is necessary to involve a physician, most usefully a child psychiatrist specialising in eating disorders. Although starving and weight issues are addressed in the individual and family therapy regularly as aspects of the collaborative relationship, the involvement of a doctor who thoroughly understands anorexia nervosa is essential in addressing medical issues connected with starvation. This is important because of the possible occurrence of death through lack of potassium contributing to a heart-attack or the occurrence of permanent physical damage or life-risking conditions connected with starvation.

Conclusion

Since children remain their parents' children throughout adulthood, the most satisfactory therapeutic outcome is achieved when parents are helped through parents' groups, couple therapy and family therapy to work with their children to repair the broken connections between the parents and their children. This enables the young person in the inevitable moments of internal and external crises to find the courage and strength to work through difficulties with the support of understanding parents rather than resorting again to anorexia nervosa which is prone to occur later in life in moments of adversity. It also means that after many years of arduous work as parents, the parents may have the privilege of celebrating the new-found hope and joys of their recovering anorectic children.

As part of the young person's psychological development in individual psychodynamic therapy it is hoped that a deep encounter between therapist and young person, and therapist and family will occur. A 'beautiful-enough' aesthetic encounter in therapy, as described in Chapter 8 (Understanding the imprisoned self), will contribute to the young person's pleasure in being alive and further the child's wish to invest in developing in therapy (Begoin, 2000). Through this there will develop a trust in the psychotherapist derived from being sufficiently protected from annihilation anxieties. This is the first step towards having a sense of identity and sense of good self-esteem, based on identification with the secure, good-enough internal figures – the mother and father. Identification with these good internal parents will facilitate a sense of being a well-formed young man or woman who can fulfil his/her desires and goals, which most probably will include establishing intimate relationships with others and using his/her capacities for mentalization and work, including work in understanding one's dreams.

This book, describing ways to release the imprisoned self, portrays work with the primitive, non-verbalized aspects of communication using my insight from observing infants coupled with spontaneous interactions using dreams, drawings, dramatizations and the use of my countertransference experiences. My hope is that these chapters will foster a deep and meaningful encounter between therapist, child and family.

Chapter 1

The theatre of the mouth

Introduction

In this chapter I shall describe show how infantile experiences are displayed in 'the theatre of the mouth' (Meltzer, 1986). Subsequently I shall present relevant clinical stories to portray the preoccupation with the non-speaking child, trying to pull words out of him/her or grab his attention and suggest how therapists need to change this stance and listen to 'the sound of silence' (Simon and Garfunkel, 1964; Lask, 2012). My focus on *Communication Beyond Words* (Magagna, 2012) encourages understanding of all aspects of the therapist's and the child's nonverbal communication.

In the beginning

In utero the baby's personality begins to be revealed. There is a consistency between the baby's personality seen in the womb and the newly born baby's personality (Piontelli, 1997). Some babies, particularly twin siblings, are delivered prematurely because of the pressure placed upon them in the crowded space of the womb. Those prematurely born babies who are placed in incubators are at risk of developing autistic traits. The sound and noise of the premature babies' unit as well as the bright lights, the infant's enclosure in the incubator and low staffing level contribute to the physiological instability of the newborns (White, 2004, p. 293). In the absence of the parents, the infants tend to self-comfort through adhesive identification manoeuvres described by Esther Bick (1964, 1968, 1986).

These primitive protections include using various organs as suction pads (Symington, 2002). Eyes fasten onto a light; the mouth sucks the thumb; the ears latch on to the sound of the buzzing machines and voices of often invisible nurses and parents. In each of these instances, the infants' organs are functioning to grip on to some object in order to cope with the great anxieties of falling to pieces, disintegrating or liquefying, or dropping into a terrifying space full of 'nameless dread' (Bion, 1962). The anxiety of being alone in the incubator can also lead to trying to hold the self together through rigidifying

DOI: 10.4324/9781003044970-2

the musculature of the body, rigid arching of the back and tightening of inner muscles, producing constipation and colic. When these primitive protections are overused, the parents' attunement to the baby and their containment of the baby's anxieties can help the baby trust the parents and then gradually shed some of these very early primitive protections against anxiety.

In a normal birth the baby is highly stressed and this birthing stress seems necessary to activate the systems that make possible breathing air and coping with 'life outside'. Once outside the womb, the baby's need for safety is primary. Essentially it is only mother's presence providing reliable, attuned, understanding caregiving that achieves this. The mother's holding of the newborn provides its place of care. Care involves meeting the three basic biological needs: mother's skin-to-skin contact ensures warmth, her breasts provide nutrition, and her arms cover baby for protection. The baby is neurologically wired to respond to this place with mother in many different ways. After feeding, the baby must sleep to establish the neural pathways that were fired.

When mother is absent, the newborn's brain feels unsafe, it perceives danger and threat to life, and its basic needs are not provided. The brain kicks in a powerful defence reaction, which first involves the baby in making a short burst of crying before stopping the crying. Then there is a lowering heart rate and temperature, and then the brain shuts down all activity, reverting to the immobilization defence, similar to that of frogs and reptiles. This looks like sleep! But it is not, and it is maintained by high levels of cortisol, which make the 'wear and tear' which is one of the primary causes of all subsequent problems from which preterm infants suffer. Because this is not actually sleep, the normal neurological pathways are not properly established. Instead, cortisol resulting from prolonged stress disrupts brain architecture, unless there is 'buffering protection of adult support'.

The presence of a good enough mother promotes the establishment of a higher level of brain development and the baby continues to approach caregivers. When bad experiences occur, the baby's brain fires more lower level defensive or avoidance pathways. Chronic bad experiences promote the defensive brain pathways which create 'wear and tear' on basic brain pathways. When the baby experiences future stresses and 'knocks in life', neural pathway failures are triggered. They later show themselves in various physiological and behavioural problems. This new understanding of the brain and its development can profoundly improve neonatal care. Mother and father's presence is an absolute requirement for optimal physical, emotional and intellectual development (Bergman, 2014).

Twenty-six percent of incubated premature infants had a positive result when screened for autistic traits. Abnormal scores correlated highly with internalized behavioural problems on the Child Behaviour Checklist and with socialization and communication deficits on the Vineland Scales. Also, in 2008, a growing body of data has pointed to an astonishing prevalence of higher order neurodevelopmental impairment by the time prematurely born children, who have been in an incubator, reach school age. In some studies, up to 50% of ex-preterm infants experience difficulties in executive functioning, as well as in the areas of attention and behaviour (Limperopoulos et al., 2008). Long-term eating difficulties can result from premature birth resulting in a hospital stay in an incubator because the normal pattern of interaction in which both infant and parent initiate and respond to mutually complementary behaviour is difficult to establish (Goldberg, 1979).

Moreover, preterm birth with weight lower than two kilograms is the most common direct cause of newborn mortality. The constant use of the 'kangaroo pouch' which includes exclusive and frequent breast-feeding in addition to skin-to-skin contact and support for the parent-infant dyad, has been shown to reduce mortality (World Health Organisation, 2014). Also, to avoid the overuse of these 'primitive protections against anxiety' Amez and Botero (2000) and others worldwide have developed the 'kangaroo method' of caring for premature babies. This method involves having a mother, father or relatives constantly holding the premature baby skin to skin while covering the baby with a warm cloth which is tied around the parent. The 'kangaroo method' of caring for the premature baby creates an increased attachment to the parents. The 'kangaroo method' also helps to stabilize the baby's breathing, oxygen saturation, heart rate and temperature (Dodd, 2004). This suggests that the baby's stress level and the need for primitive protections against anxiety are thus decreased.

The penumbra baby

At times there have been previous miscarriages or a twin has died in utero. Giving birth and mourning simultaneously create conflictual emotional experiences and doctors have often been heard to say, 'Celebrate the existence of your live baby! That is what you need to do now.' But the parents' emotional receptivity is impeded by the birth of the new baby, blocking the ability to mourn the loss of the dead baby (Reid, 2013). If one twin baby dies, it is often difficult to develop an attachment to the other baby. The 'penumbra baby' is the term Marguerite Reid (2013, p. 9) uses because 'the attachment between the mother and her dead infant often appears to be so strong that it can possibly leave the new baby in an area of obscurity and uncertainty that the mother finds hard to explore'.

Professionals' inattention to the parents' grief when one twin dies may delay the parents' attachment to the surviving twin. It seems important that parents be encouraged to mourn the lost child appropriately by talking about the infant, naming the baby, holding a memorial service, and openly expressing their grief. The ungrieved baby's death can function as a shadow over the newly born baby's existence and leave the live baby filled with the parents' anxiety about the baby's survival ... for years to come! Reid (2013) suggests that when the mothers have suffered the loss of a concurrent loss of another baby, the live baby, 'the penumbra baby', often overuses primitive protections such as avoidance of eye contact, not snuggling up, back arching and pulling away from the mother's feeding and touch. Also the 'penumbra baby's' overuse of primitive protections often results in feeding difficulties.

Normal expectations for the birth of a baby

We assume that a baby is born, looks into the eyes of the mother, turns to find the familiar voice of the father saying hello. The baby anticipates that there will be feeding, emotionally nurturing and protective parents. In the first few minutes the baby is already so observant. One father, rather excited to be greeting his baby born a few minutes previously, stuck his tongue out and after a brief second the baby stuck his tongue out in return, copying his father's facial gesture.

The baby has a repertoire to signal to the parents to come. The baby cries out when distressed, hungry, angry, in pain. Simultaneously the baby beckons the parents by waving extended arms, This is usually accompanied by baby kicking rapidly.

Through the couple's union an emotional cradle for the baby is created. There can be a complex weaving of this cradle depending on the personalities of each of the parents and their identifications with their internalised parents.

Internalised parents

Peter Fonagy and Mary Target (1997) have suggested that the nature of the baby's attachment relationship to each parental figure can be significantly different. A baby's secure attachment to a parent is related to a caregiver's capacity for receiving the child's intolerable feelings and modulating them through containment described by Bion. If one parent is defensive and one responsive to the child, the child will internalise both an insecure attachment which interferes with mental development and a secure attachment which promotes the child's capacity for mentalisation. Therefore, we cannot afford to hold onto Winnicott's statement 'There is no baby without a mother' (1964). This is a seriously inaccurate misrepresentation, interfering with how we assist a child to develop. In fact, there is no baby without a mother and a father! The father's capacity for containment either assists or interferes with the baby's psychological and intellectual development!

The baby's personality is already developing in utero (Piontelli, 1989) and 'Ghosts in the Nursery' (Fraiberg et al., 1980) suggests that different unconscious trans-generational factors affect the parents' parenting of a child. The couple's cradle of emotion supporting one another and the newborn generates the child's love, trust and hope. The parents' hostility, depression and insecure attachment can leave the child with no space in the parent's psyche in which to project 'nameless dread' and anxiety. In a hostile couple interaction, the baby's eyes flit fearfully between one parent and the other. The absence of the 'couple's cradle for the baby' (Magagna and Piercey, 2020) promotes the baby's hate, frustration, anxiety, despair and often accompanying eating difficulties.

The theatre of the mouth

As Spitz (1955) has described, the oral cavity of the mouth is a central part of the mother and baby's physical and emotional relationship. Weekly infant observations provide a unique, naturalistic way of understanding the connection between mouth/nipple and mind and the accompanying phantasies. Brief infant observation vignettes will convey four aspects of the baby's relationship to the mother. These infant observations will be used to elucidate similar states of mind present in the child/therapist relationship and be followed by therapeutic ways of relating to 'the troubled infant in the child'.

First infant observation: the collapsed crying mouth – giving up

Baby Jon, aged two months

Father is in full time work and mother has resumed three weekly 12-hour shifts as a telephonist. Jon becomes more fretful being left with the baby-sitter. Simultaneously, and conceivably both because of her work and his crying which overwhelms her, mother begins regularly to leave Jon, when he awakens in the night crying, to comfort himself or cry himself to sleep.

On one occasion mother leaves Jon in his room, crying so loudly and for so long that he begins to choke and gasp for air. Arriving to check on him, mother says, 'I don't want Jon to cry too long,' but it has already been 'too long'. Terrified, Jon clenches his fists and tries to use his legs to push himself up from his bed. He is trying to get out of this terrible position of lying helpless on the bed, a miserable baby left without his external mother and also without a good internal mother. In lieu of this he is relying on the clenching of his fingers to hold together his Self, which he fears is 'falling to pieces'. Jon's precocious agility becomes a necessity as he attempts to use his legs to push himself out of the position of being a 'helpless, wretched left-alone baby'.

A vicious cycle seems to be initiated: in identification with her own mother, mother leaves Jon for even longer periods; Jon becomes more distressed; as a result, mother becomes more persecuted. This results in mother increasingly detaching herself from Jon, prompting Jon to cry alone for even longer periods. Jon's fragile 'bridge to mother' is gradually being broken. Jon alienates himself by replacing her with his own body and sticking to objects as a protection against overwhelming terrors. Jon's anger with his mother leads to further fragility of his internal mother. This internal situation of having only a frightening, damaged internal mother creates in Jon a terrifying anxiety. He experiences nightmarish images instead of a good internal mother (O'Shaughnessy, 1964).

Fonagy tells us that:

> The reactions of children under stress have their origins in the parents' defensive strategies. Many of the shortcomings in the parents' responsiveness to their child's needs derive from their own defences against acknowledging and understanding similar negative affect in themselves. The parents' defences have their origin in their own developmental history and in turn make it difficult for them to respond empathically to affective signals from their infant. Because the infant cannot rely on the parents sufficiently to respond to his signals of negative affective states and thereby to reduce them, he must find alternative ways to diminish them.
>
> (Fonagy et al., 1993, p. 8)

Without a good psychic apparatus, a good internal mother, the infant will resort to adhesive mechanisms to hold self together or dissociate.

As time progresses, we see Jon hurting himself.

Jon, seven months

Jon takes some keys and one by one he puts them in his mouth. He puts the long keys so far back in his throat that they occasionally make him gag. He makes an expression of distaste as he samples each key. After five minutes of this play, he pokes the key hard into the back of his throat and breaks into a sob. Jon seems identified with an internalised intrusive and hurtful object when he repeatedly hurts himself on this occasion.

At two years, Jon's emotional development remained a concern. He frequently switched on the television and glued himself to it while switching off his connection to the family. He became increasingly involved with hard objects like keys, a block, a screwdriver. Jon seemed to almost encapsulate his 'hidden tears of grief' (S. Klein 1980) for he did not facilitate the parents' containment of his emotional states. Mother began to share with the observer her worry about Jon's poor emotional development as reflected in his very noticeable delay in using language.

Jon had given up beckoning through crying and beckoning through talking. It is as though certain aspects of Jon's mouth disappeared from Jon's point of view, along with an image of a mother to whom he could turn (Winnicott 1963, p. 222). Turned away from mother, Jon clung onto the activities he could do with his toy drill and toolbox, Jon was alone with his hidden grief. His hidden grief was symbolised by his difficulties with eating.

Grief underlying eating difficulties can be hidden through achievement as well as through using toy drills and a toolbox. A 17-year-old girl played the cello eight hours a day, then suddenly we see her here.

Example of giving up: emaciated Yufang, aged 17

Emaciated, eyes closed to every object or person, she lay on the hospital bed. She opened her mouth to neither food nor drink and seemed not to notice anything including urine trickling out of her. With her straight dark hair and smooth oval Modigliani face, she looked like a porcelain doll. Yufang was motionless throughout the day and night. When after some time she began to respond, she treated any nurse's touch or word like a mosquito creating a stinging irritation. She looked as though the umbilical cord that held her in life had been broken. There seemed to be no emotional point to her existence. Like the 17 other young people I have seen for psychotherapy, Yufang had felt so profoundly helpless and hopeless she had pervasively retreated from life, not walking, talking or eating. Yufang gave herself up to death because of overwhelming cumulative trauma punctuated by some significant traumas.

In the initial phase of therapy, while Yufang was primarily lifeless and verbally mute, it seemed necessary for me to use my heart, my body, my soul to help her gather her whole being together 'to be emotionally present' in the room. I described a mood that I felt in the room: good to be her together, suspicious of me, curious about what I will say, how she glanced at me. Using my infant observation capacities, I greeted each of her nonverbal gestures. I sometimes experienced an image of a turtle gradually being born and sufficiently integrated to gradually peep out of an impermeable shell and then disappearing back inside the darkness. My feeling emotionally present and using words of understanding were vital in evoking Yufang's wish to gather together her apparently disintegrated emotional and mental functioning again, and depart from her dark world of 'not-thinking' and eat.

Second infant observation: baby's mouth in battle of omnipotent control

Baby Bobby, aged three and a half months

Mother anxiously holds baby, who is serious as he looks at his hand and rotates it in front of his eyes. With his left hand he then grasps his right wrist and brings his fist to his mouth. Saliva bubbles are coming out of his mouth. Baby then sucks his tightly closed fist. Six or seven times his mother takes baby's hand from his mouth and baby returns his fist firmly to his mouth. When mother shows baby the bottle, he looks at it as though he doesn't recognize it. He then quickly turns away and looks at his rotating fist. This happens regularly when the bottle is offered to him.

As mother approaches with the bottle, baby Bobby quickly inserts his fist in his mouth again. Mother pushes baby's hand away from his mouth and inserts the teat. Bobby sucks once and quickly spits out the teat and with it the milk. Each time this sequence is repeated, mother becomes increasingly forceful and insistent as she firmly presses the bottle into baby's mouth.

Baby grasps the bottle with both hands, pushes it away and spits out all the milk from his mouth. Mother becomes more nervy, intrusive, and angry and baby Bobby becomes increasingly strong-willed and persecuted as he wrenches the bottle out of his mouth, vomits out the milk and returns to sucking his fist.

Mother is panicked because she knows she needs to feed baby to keep him alive. She is also angry and frustrated by her sense of impotence. Baby has retreated from the external mother and is in some way imagining himself to be a 'baby inside mother' omnipotently feeding himself with his fist.

An anxious, irritated insecurely attached mother who has not developed reflective functioning (Slade, 2007) resorts to control rather than spontaneous attunement in the caregiving of her baby. The baby feels intruded upon and persecuted as the battle over who owns the entry to the mouth ensues. He refuses mother's food.

Clinical example: Jane, with anorexia nervosa, aged 14

Jane wasn't told that she was being admitted into the inpatient unit. Her parents were afraid of what she would do if she knew beforehand. When Jane came with a strong, defiant stride into the therapy room, she averted her gaze and went to the window, where she stood with her hard back firmly positioned to keep me out. Her face, covered with long, blonde hair, was invisible through the session as she looked out of the window. I had to use my countertransference experiences to voice different states of mind reflected in the tautness of Jane's back musculature, the movements of her head, the rhythm of her barely visible gestural changes. In our eating disorder inpatient unit we realized that putting up a barrier suggests that there is a mind present. There is a Self healthier than Yufang's, for at least Jane is able to fight when terrified and or angry. This is part of her anorexic stance towards food.

Third infant observation: the gaping mouth present in over-attunement

Fraiberg et al. (1980) describe how despite intense love for the child, a parent can identify with internalized ghosts of the past now residing internally. Here is an example of a mother trying to be the best mother she can possibly be to her baby. She attunes to her baby's every wish, as we see here.

Baby Susan, ten months

Baby is sitting in the stroller, eating cracker bits. She watches an ant crawl on her arm and pinches it between her fingers. Mother notices this ant and asks, 'What's that?' and goes back to folding the laundry. Baby turns the cracker bag upside down, spilling some of the crackers onto the floor. Mother helps the baby to set the bag upright, but baby spills the crackers again. Mother takes her out of the stroller and baby lifts one arm and mother says, 'Oh, you want me to carry you to the other room,' and mother proceeds to do this. They play ball in the living room. Later, baby pulls at the front of Mother's blouse. Mother says, 'Okay, you want some milk.' Mother offers her breast to baby. Baby latches on to nurse while squeezing Mother's other breast with her hand. Mother takes baby's hand away from her breast and holds her hand. This action is repeated several times.

Mother is perfectly attuned to baby's wishes, but she seems unable to acknowledge baby's aggression towards the breast that isn't in her mouth, she is not able to acknowledge baby's anger towards her for departing to do the laundry, thus dropping baby from her attentive vision, rather than staying with her. Mother has also not felt any incentive to gradually wean baby from the breast-feeding for fear baby would protest. Baby walks around with an open mouth when not at the breast. Sometimes saliva oozes out of the sides of her mouth. Mother attunes to the baby, but cannot provide what Winnicott (Padel, 1987, p. 273) calls 'a continuum of care' in which she gradually faces the baby's protest about her separations from baby. Baby has not been able to have a mother receiving her protests and thus not able to internalise a containing mother. There remains simply 'a gaping hole': where the breast was in the mouth. Mother and baby have not fully separated. Baby has not elaborated upon the frustrations of separation from the mother. Baby has no speech, mother anticipates baby's wishes, and occasionally baby uses her hands to signal to mother. Baby tends to turn to food as a method of avoiding anxiety.

In some instances, when the mother has not been able to separate from the baby fearing the baby's hostility, unable to bear the baby's pain, the baby does not exercise her own identity, find her own 'mouth-self', does not bite, does not call out, does not experience a self that is required to struggle for what she wants. Here we see the consequences in this clinical vignette.

Sam, a three-year-old eating disordered autistic child in family therapy

When breast-feeding was terminated, Sam, like other babies I have known, had convulsions. The depressed mother, who had had a miscarriage, felt very guilty about the weaning, which was accompanied by Sam's convulsions and thenceforth she acquiesced to any demand made by Sam. The father, in negative identification with his own violent, sexually abusive father, was unable to place any limits on Sam or on the mother/child sleeping together. Like the vignette above, he has not found his 'mouth-self', does not bite, does not want to chew food, does not call out to the parents to struggle for what he wants. When Sam felt he was misunderstood he pulled out his own hair. Avoiding his parents' gaze, turning away from his parents and their food and not developing language, suggested that Sam's relationship with his attentive parents was impeded.

I helped Sam and encouraged his parents to help him play games which included toppling objects, tearing paper, shouting 'hurt' or 'cross', stamping his feet, banging on pots, shouting 'away' to a playmate when he was being annoyed. They had to say the words for him, but they were giving him ways of thinking about experiences with words rather than hair-pulling. In the sessions I used ways of transforming his crossness involving hair-pulling into one of one of these other methods. He no longer inhibited his biting and he gradually he began eating that involved biting solid foods.

With Sam, I describe the eating disordered child's relationships to sensory objects and the use of sensory experiences in relation to self and therapist. Here is an example.

When the stuffed dog is thrown down, I vary the pitch, loudness and quality of my voice to echo the emotion and sensory experience of throwing the dog: 'Goodbye Johnny' is said in a loud, quick and somewhat harsh way a way, which is attuned to the force and velocity of Sam's throwing of the dog. 'Hello Johnny' is spoken by me in a soft, gentle way as Sam puts his dog in my lap.

With my mouth I speak in identification with Sam and acknowledge as precisely as possible the nature of feeling present in each gesture Sam makes. I also personify the object with which he is playing, stating what it would feel like if the object were a person in relation to Sam. I am entering Sam's dream world in which phantasies underlie each of his hand gestures (Isaacs, 1948). 'Greeting Sam's gestures' with my wonderings enables Sam to reach down to aspects of his inner life that have previously been unknown, nameless, frightening and chaotic. Some of his present emotions will certainly contain aspects of emotions of Sam's experience in his preverbal infancy. Sam's gestures are filled with conversation about his mental life.

There were various ways Sam was helped to eat: I discovered ways of receiving and understanding his parents' feelings and their hostility about their own unmet needs during family therapy sessions. I assisted them to acknowledge and bear Sam's hostility and tolerate his extreme frustration when they did not do things 'his way'. Together we observed Sam, acknowledged his terror, repressed rage, and other inhibited feelings including jealousy of his parents having time alone at night. This allowed the emergence of a little boy who was affectionate to his parents. They were encouraged by me to take photos of Sam and his dog Johnny and make books with stories they wrote about him and illustrated with photos. They left these books for him to look at during the day and the evening when alone.

By the end of the year of family therapy, Sam developed more language and was describing some of his feelings via his stuffed animal, his dog, Johnny: 'bumped head' and 'sad' followed by 'no Sam'. The parents were thrilled for it seemed that Sam had internalised our way of receiving and thinking about his feelings, and he was now speaking and doing the same verbally for his dog, Johnny. After one year of therapy Sam spoke with more words, showed aggression outwards, rather than pulling his hair and gradually he opened his mouth to an adequate amount of food. Through therapy he was able to grow psychologically and physically as a normal child who tolerated eating at mealtimes with his parents.

Fourth infant observation: playing possum – the terrified mouth

This fourth example of an Indian baby, Acchal, will be followed by psychotherapy sessions with a girl who is now 11 years old. I have acknowledged important issues in the parent-child relationship, but perhaps we are failing to look more closely at how sibling relationships can provoke the second-born baby's use of 'autistic-like protections against anxiety'. Here we see Virat, aged 23 months, who is triangulated into the marital relationship and paired with mother, as though he is mother's special partner during the day when the father is away. As we subsequently see, this unconscious pairing has a powerful influence on how mother protects her daughter, Acchal.

Acchal, five months and Virat, 23 months

Acchal is sitting on mother's lap, facing outwards. Mother is holding the end of a bottle positioned in her mouth. Acchal has both hands circled around the top of the bottle as she sucks the milk. Virat approaches Acchal with a dummy. Mother says, 'Acchal is drinking her milk now and she doesn't want the dummy.' Ignoring Mother's words, Virat swiftly thrusts the dummy into Acchal's mouth. Mother admonishes, 'Don't do that!' but Mother does not use her hands to physically stop Virat. Vaun continues to force the dummy into Acchal's mouth until the teat of the bottle is pushed out. In response, Acchal whimpers and bursts into cries.

Virat cries out in protest when mother takes the pacifier out of Acchal's mouth. Mother then turns Acchal outwards so that she is leaning on mother's chest and re-seated her on her lap. Acchal looks stupefied, with her eyes glazed over and unfocused. Her fists are tightly closed, but the rest of her body is limp. Virat pushes Acchal to the side as he gets on mother's lap then gets down and goes to his playroom. Meanwhile, Acchal remains motionless while continuing to stare in a dissociated state into space.

When Mother returns the bottle nipple to Acchal's mouth, she doesn't close her mouth, doesn't suck. Milk dribbles out of her mouth. Mother tries to reinsert the nipple. Milk again dribbles out of Acchal's still mouth. Mother gives up the feeding. With her eyes still blank and unfocused, Acchal rocks back and forth in an autistic-like rhythm.

There are repeated interactions in which Virat interferes with Acchal's relationship with mother. Nine months later, still not having recovered from Acchal's arrival into the family, Virat is still pushing Acchal off the chair, taking her possessions, and demanding mother be with him to the exclusion of Acchal. The regularity of this type of interaction between the siblings may produce an internalised attack, represented by the internalised brother, on an empathic connection with mother. Also, Acchal's sense of being unloved and unprotected by mother develops. She often rejects mother's food.

The excessive use of these protections in infancy may mask an underlying 'basic fault' in the child's developing personality (Balint, 1968). Then a huge regression can occur when ten to 11-year-old sexual development is beginning and the child is entering the stage of moving from family to peer group relationships.

The encapsulated selective eater

In trying to be present for a young child using primitive omnipotence, there are only two feelings: love and fear (Leunig, 1990). Fear can stop the child from loving and eating. As a child utilising primitive omnipotence is developing psychologically and beginning to form a trusting relationship with an adult, he often draws or describes a sensation of the self with feelings being imprisoned inside a structure like a castle, jail or tower.

Clinical example: eating disordered Acchal, ten years

As her pubertal body started changing and she faced the challenges of being involved more with her peer group, Acchal, although academically continuing her written work, became completely mute at school and intensified her selective eating at home. When Acchal entered therapy, her Indian trainee psychotherapist suffered the anguish of feeling she was a bad therapist if Acchal didn't talk to her. I suggested that her task was not to make Acchal talk, her task was to understand Acchal's emotions. The therapist felt extremely anxious also about her therapy being considered 'no good' by the impatient parents wanting 'a quick fix'. A hatred of feeling impotent, the fear of being rejected by both the child and the parents and the anxiety about being criticized by me, her supervisor, invaded the trainee psychotherapist's mind.

An early session with Acchal

Acchal didn't look at the therapist as she said hello and walked hesitatingly into the room. After a few moments, she sat down at the table. She didn't reach for anything, but looked at a piece of paper. The therapist asked Acchal if she wanted to draw and she nodded 'yes'. The therapist handed her a sheet of paper and Acchal folded it into the shape of a rectangular container. Somewhat later she reached for the coloured markers and drew a very colourful abstract design with matching coloured swirls on it.

Then she made four coloured triangles in the corners. When Acchal left the session, the therapist said 'goodbye', but Acchal walked out without looking at her, without even a nod acknowledging a goodbye.

Reviewing the session, the trainee therapist said, 'I felt very anxious, over-whelmed by this feeling of not knowing what I am doing, not knowing how to help her, feeling very inadequate. I am trying to feel comfortable with the silence.' As the therapist spoke, I was aware that I had to help her feel she could think aloud and didn't need to ask questions, but could make ongoing comments which described Acchal's gestures of being afraid to grasp, her finding the courage to grasp the colours and how while being with the therapist she was letting her hands be free with the colour.

A middle session with mute, selective eating Acchal

Subsequently there was a funny scene in the corridor in which a man was yawning while making a funny snorting noise. Acchal and her therapist looked at one another and when they entered the room the therapist laughed a little and Acchal pursed her lips so hard she actually couldn't manage. She turned red trying so hard not to burst out laughing! The therapist suggests, 'It's so hard not to laugh out loud with me. I can see how much you want to!'

Acchal looked at the therapist, trying to compose herself, but it was hard. She continued to purse her lips, but she was still chuckling inside. Acchal needed the therapist to acknowledge, 'Poor Acchal, she wants to laugh and isn't allowed to laugh.'

Acchal then sealed her lips tightly and picked up some pipe cleaners and began making something. After a few minutes, the therapist asked her, 'What are you making?' Acchal turned to her, look into her eyes, and for one of the first times she answered, 'A necklace.' The therapist could have said, 'Brave Acchal, you defied those "hard lips" that won't let you be with me.' When the therapist stopped talking, Acchal pursed her lips but she did not cover her mouth as she sometimes did.

We see here how Acchal is conflicted: now there is a self that feels sponta-neously joined to the therapist and feels like laughing with her, but there is also this 'hard self' that is completely against opening up and becoming intimate with her therapist. These 'hard lips' are being used to protect the soft, vulner-able self that has been so hurt and rejected in the past and they remain hard to protect Acchal from her being disappointed and hurt by the therapist. Acchal needs the therapist to acknowledge, 'Something is hard, trying to protect you. It won't let you laugh with me.'

In a later part of the session, feeling a bit more trusting of the therapist, Acchal answered her question, but after she quickly snapped her lips back together, as though she must not want anything from the therapist, must not desire to speak with her for fear of being rejected, but she now had the courage to respond at this moment.

A psychotherapist lacking a secure attachment to her helpmate, psychoanalysis, may stop interpreting anything about the transference/countertransference rela-tionship between the child and the therapist. A stalemate can then occur. The therapist is having to wonder within herself asking, how did this feel? What is the emotional issue now between us when this blanking occurs?

A later session with Acchal

Acchal takes out a starfish drawing. The therapist suggests that maybe she (the therapist) looks up on her iPhone just a little more information about the starfish. Acchal stares at the therapist in an interested way. This is the first time the therapist has ever suggested such a thing. The therapist says, 'The starfish are covered in armour. If a creature bites off a part it can regenerate a limb.' Acchal's face is very expressive as the therapist expresses her wonder and interest in the starfish. She goes back to drawing her starfish. The therapist says, 'Some people imagine themselves to be a specific animal. I wonder if you feel a bit like a starfish ... as though you feel like you need some armour to get through here.' Acchal stares at the therapist blankly and draws eyes and a smile on the starfish. The therapist says, 'That looks like a friendly starfish for even with its armour it is smiling.'

As the session is very near the end, Acchal draws a hedgehog. The therapist talks about how the fur at the top of the hedgehog is like a protective spine, prickly, and the fur on the tummy is very soft. The therapist adds that when the hedgehog is scared it rolls itself up into a tight ball and the prickly spines protect it from the predators. For Acchal, who tightly closes her lips to avoid smiling or laughing at times in the session, this is an opening of the relationship with the therapist, Acchal experiences an emerging friendliness towards the therapist who understands her fears. The problem is, having felt so rejected earlier by Acchal's blank look, the therapist can't bear the idea of being rejected again if she acknowledges Acchal's appreciation of the therapist as shown by the starfish's smile and eyes looking at the therapist. When the trainee therapist holds such a strong sense of being rejected by non-speaking, selective eating Acchal, it is difficult for her to realize that Acchal may also feel she is having to 'curl up with her prickly spine' for protection as she leaves the protective space of the therapy.

When parents and therapist have felt rejected for so long by a child who does not express affection, it may be a shock to let their own 'starfish armour' melt in order to accept and directly receive the child's smile and attentive look. In fact, as Acchal began emerging from her armour the mother wrote:

> Acchal has begun saying to me:
> 'I love you mummy'
> 'You are my best friend'...
> 'You are pretty'...
> 'You are so nice'...
> At times, also, unusually, Acchal is becoming weepy.

It is possible to begin to understand that selective eating often involves hostility and subsequent persecution by parental figures, which gets projected onto certain foods and the therapist. Not-speaking in therapy can often accompany eating difficulties.

Rosenfeld (2012) suggests that encapsulation is used to preserve infantile healthy bonds with the mother. Preserving the good links with the internalised mother may involve impeding connections between mouth and an intrusive, unresponsive, depressed or emotionally disturbed mother, and avoidance of food is the result. After some psychotherapy, still being silent, eating disordered Acchal was finally able to reveal through her drawing that within her prison-cell of silence she felt herself to be crying. Her hard omnipotent back was protecting her from her mother who was looking between the cell bars trying to be with her.

Simultaneously, Acchal was experiencing a vicious debate between two conflicting emotions: her love of being understood versus her fear of being touched emotionally by someone she feared would let her down. Later in therapy, when she began talking, she described how when she felt criticized or in conflict with someone she imagined herself in a bomb-shelter with its hard walls. Acchal felt herself go into a very hard state where no one could reach her and she could not bear to eat. The bad part about it was also that she also couldn't reach herself and know what she was feeling and that was frightening.

The importance of parent work accompanying individual psychotherapy

As a mother of a 'cut-off encapsulated child', one might feel at some point experience an intense wish for intimacy to develop with her child. She might be ecstatic about the child's emerging vocalised wish for closeness. However, if a mother is herself encapsulated with a limited capacity for the reception of intense emotional infantile states, she may feel threatened or oppressed by Acchal's 'mother hunger' which emerges in the course of therapy.

After Acchal began speaking again, such is the case with Acchal's mother who says, 'My child is too absorbed in me. I feel so persecuted by her.' Mother's fragile personality is becoming destabilized by the Acchal's wish for intimacy. It felt safer when Acchal was more encapsulated, as previously described. At this point Mother accepted that the couple needed to do some parental work to bear the possessive longing of their daughter who was slowly emerging from her 'starfish armour'.

What is interesting is that mother is so detached from the father as a source of support at this turbulent time of changing relationships. It is for this reason that I suggest that we as professionals should be thinking of the couple, father and mother, as 'the cradle of emotional support' for each other (Magagna and Piercey, 2020). Parental work accompanying the child in individual therapy is essential. As the non-eating or selectively eating child progresses in therapy there is revealed a previously entrapped vulnerable self with an intense need and longing for emotional nurturance and understanding. Parental work is particularly crucial for the child relinquishing autistic protections to survive and turn towards the security provided by the parents.

The therapist's attempt to pull words out of the patient

The therapist's anxiety about progress being slow can lead to a shift from the therapist's secure attachment to the psychoanalytic method to the therapist's use of control: trying to teach words to a speech-delayed, eating disordered child, asking a lot of questions to get the child to talk, thinking speech therapy is the answer. Pushing and controlling the child replaces the psychoanalytic method of greeting the gestures and realising that the eating disordered child is communicating states of mind through these gestures. If the therapist has a secure attachment to the psychoanalytic method, and trusts it to do all that it can, then the therapist will receive the child's nonverbal communication, observe how it resonates within herself, and provide understanding rather than searching for ways to make the child speak.

The therapist bearing being rejected

When a therapist speaks and faces the child's blank eyes, blank expression, and closed mouth, there are several possibilities:

- It may be because the therapist is completely off track and the child ignores the therapist
- Or it may be that the child has attacked the therapist's entry with a new thought and a barrier is established through blanking
- Or it may be that in the countertransference the therapist is having to repeatedly bear being the rejected one, the useless one, the unloved one, the one angry about an unresponsive object.

We need to remember that while the mouth may be barricading thoughts from being spoken to the therapist, the unconscious still has ears, still has a mind that can hear the therapist, and it may or may not be attacking the possibility of thinking about what the therapist is saying.

Being a psychotherapist with a child requires me to frequently question to find what impediments to experiencing painful loss of intimacy and rejection may reside within oneself. One needs time and emotional space to examine one's own mental state in working with a child. It is essential to give birth to one's own inner child, to find the space to get to know the truth of one's own emotional experience, to form a picture of how one feels and to then find nourishment and protection for my own inner child. This is necessary also for both the mother and the father.

Ultimately, the more the therapist pulls for words or drawings or attention from the child, the more tightly shut the mouth to food and the child's mind can become. As a therapist one begins to recognise that a relationship is not about receiving looks or words or drawings from the child, rather it is about the child finding his own wish to reach out to the other. As a therapist one freely offers oneself to another, to find meaning together, to understand impediments to forming a good rapport with each other.

A child's words may be helpful to the therapist and speaking to the child can be useful, but words may not be the essential ingredient to helping a child with an eating difficulty. It is the inner openness, the state of the souls in relation to one another, which is the most important therapeutic ingredient. The 'theatre of the mouth' dramatizes the child's emotional state in relation to the therapist. When the child begins to open both his mouth to speaking and eating and his mind, the therapist and the family require the emotional capacity to greet the arrival of the child's very needy, very dependent, extremely vulnerable infantile state of mind. Healing both the child's difficulties in eating and difficulties in speaking in therapy also involve bearing the brunt of the child's infantile hostility aroused by feeling rejected during the therapist's mis-attunements and separations from the child. This therapeutic work is more fully described in *The Silent Child: Communication Without Words* (Magagna, 2012).

Chapter 2

Ways of assessing children with severe eating difficulties

> When I'm thin I'll be happy – I'm fat and therefore unhappy. My body is huge and disgusting. Nobody tries to understand who I really am. They are only interested in how much I weigh and how they can make me fatter.

These words, spoken by an anorectic girl after the failure of a treatment programme for young people with anorexia, underline the importance of having as assessment process which enables a child to feel that the whole of her being, her feelings, her physical condition, her body sensations, her thoughts, are accepted and understood. I have heard similar words spoken by anorectic young people from many cultures around the world: Russian, South American, Chinese, Indian, Polish, French, Italian, South African, Australian. Feeling fat and not understood is a kind of mantra spoken by anorectic young people everywhere.

Underlying hypothesis

My hypothesis is that refusal to eat does not simply refer to refusing to open the mouth to take in food. It might simultaneously mean closing the mind to the emotional experience of oneself and others. 'I won't eat' can in fact signify closing the mind in the face of conflicts or withdrawing from the nurturing emotional link with the mother. The anorectic child's fear of being fat, as well as being linked to the pressure society exerts on young women to become thin, also includes the fear of bodily sensations and intense emotions that overwhelm the child to the point of threatening her sense of identity, her perception of the form and size of her body and her own mental health (Palazzoli, 1978).

Many anorectic young people have a distorted image of their own body, actually perceiving it visually and sensually as larger than it is in reality (Farrell, 1995). Such perceptions are also manifested fleetingly at moments of experiencing intense emotion. Dieting, and thus attaining control of the shape of the body, is initially a relief to the child, for she no longer feels a 'helpless victim' of bodily sensations and emotions, but rather she feels an active and potent agent (Garner and Garfinkel, 1997). Starving can induce a state of

DOI: 10.4324/9781003044970-3

euphoria as well as a sense of not being a slave to her own desires. The potent, active self has a sense of being in control, through using 'mental dieting' which restricts the awareness of threatening feelings and bodily sensations. The child's lack of a strong and effective internal psychic structure, which normally develops from the experience of being understood by parents, creates the necessity to resort to denial to interrupt contact with more profound emotional life that is frightening, overwhelming or sad. Meeting and getting to know a child for the first time can be intimidating for a child with these characteristics. One often finds a physically withdrawn child using a 'mask' of silence or a superficial response such as a nervous smile that hides a more serious underlying psychopathology.

Often the anorectic child is reliant on an internal 'prison guard', a self-protective force which restricts the intake of food, threatens her when she speaks with the therapist and promises an artificial paradise in exchange for avoiding conflictual and painful emotional experiences. However, the 'prison guard' also prevents the experiencing of pleasurable moments and intimate relationships (Magagna, 1998).

This well-concealed prison guard is similar to a drug which substitutes itself for relationships with other people in the external world. It involves a type of omnipotent self-sufficiency, in identification with a sort of 'super-parent figure' which protects the child from becoming 'too fat', too full of intense feelings and infantile anxieties arising in intimate relationships with family members or peers (Rosenfeld, 1987a).

The assessment and formulation of a treatment plan

The context in which evaluation and psychotherapy take place is crucial. The therapeutic structure which I have found most effective includes the following:

- At least two diagnostic meetings with the family to understand the difficulties and strengths of the family members, the family pattern of interaction and shared family conflicts.
- An individual assessment to ascertain the individual psychopathology underlying the eating disturbance, bearing in mind that the anorectic child and the bulimic child have different typical modes of behaviour with specific functions in relation to the family dynamics which conceal a wide range of emotional difficulties.
- An assessment by a doctor, or preferably a child psychiatrist, experienced in eating disorders who remains aware of the ongoing treatment process and can regularly monitor the child's weight, perform blood tests and discuss the child's physical well-being with both the child and the parents.
- Making a plan for contemporaneous therapeutic work with the parents alone and the family accompanying the individual therapy. This helps the child and offers the parents or the family a secure context in which they are

able to explore problematic aspects of their relationship with the child and develop and utilize their own capacities to understand and help one another.

- Consideration of the possibility of a hospital admission if the child is or becomes seriously unwell. This is particularly important to consider for those severely ill patients when they are facing the first holiday separation from the therapist (see Chapter 3 on individual psychotherapy).

Types of eating disorders

In order to create the most adequate treatment plan, it is helpful to identify the specific type of eating disorder. Some of the main eating disorders are as follows:

Anorexia nervosa. This is found in children from the age of seven. The diagnosis is based on the following criteria:

- The refusal of food.
- Weight loss or failure to gain weight during the period of pre-adolescent growth in the absence of any physical or other mental illness.
- Two or more of the following symptoms:

  - preoccupation with body weight
  - preoccupation with the consumption of calories
  - distorted body image
  - fear of fatness
  - self-induced vomiting
  - intensive physical activity
  - laxative abuse or purging (Lask, 1993).

Bulimia nervosa. This problem, more typically found among adolescents and adults, is less frequent in children under 14. 'Bulimia nervosa' refers to a cyclical behaviour in which the refusal of food alternates with uncontrolled eating followed by self-induced vomiting, often accompanied by the abuse of laxatives (Russell, 1985). The psychological process underlying this behaviour includes an unbridled greed and a subsequent wish to free the body from the food that has turned into rubbish through the process of having been voraciously devoured at difficult moments.

Food avoidance emotional disorder (FAED), selective eating and food refusal. These disturbances are not accompanied by the characteristic preoccupation with body size, shape and weight. Instead, emotional factors lead to a determined avoidance of specific foods, all food, or food in selective situations, for example at school. Medical investigation is advisable, to exclude the possibility of a tumour preventing the experience of hunger, or the possibility of another physical illness preventing weight gain.

Pervasive retreat (PAWS) (Nunn et al., 2014). The child presents as underweight, adamantly rejecting food and drink and being unable to walk or talk, to eat or drink. At times the child remains virtually immobile in a curled up position of withdrawal from acknowledgement of external stimuli. Certain hysterical features and post-traumatic stress responses and depressive or psychotic disorders may be present underneath this symptom of pervasive retreat.

Loss of appetite as a consequence of depression or psychosis. In a study conducted by Fosson et al. (1987) almost half of 48 children with early onset anorexia were considered to be moderately or severely depressed. The loss of appetite and food refusal is sometimes linked to psychotic anxieties about food. When appetite loss is a consequence of depression or psychotic thinking, the preoccupation with weight or the shape of the body is often absent.

Criteria for evaluating the risk of suicide

Since many children with eating difficulties show secretiveness and massive denial, it is difficult to evaluate the risk of suicide and the gravity of accompanying depression and anxiety associated with underlying psychotic, borderline or neurotic psychopathology. If the child is too old to play, it can be helpful to encourage her to describe dreams which may convey phantasies and fears about which she is unable to speak directly (Natterson, 1980).

The risk of suicide warranting protective measures in relation to the child is signalled by a combination of the following factors:

- There is an apparently unmodifiable sadomasochistic relationship between the child and people such as parents who are important to her.
- The parents feel persecuted by the child's eating difficulties and are very critical in their relationship with her.
- The dreams contain some basic themes of death, destructiveness towards the self or other persons, or images that represent the sensation of being trapped, struggling unsuccessfully, or giving up and going away peacefully from the primary figure.
- The risk of suicide is always present when the anorectic child, freed from some defensive strategies during the assessment or in the course of treatment, attempts to face such emotions as sadness, desperation or a sense of severe persecutory guilt or depression. Included in that which follows are five types of suicidal phantasies (Campbell and Hale, 2017), with material taken from my clinical work.

Phantasy of fusion: A 14-year-old anorectic girl was very disappointed because she had been discharged from hospital; returning home she dreamt of floating into the clouds and meeting God, with whom she engaged in a non-stop conversation. No one else was present. When I discussed this dream with her, she revealed that she would soon die because she had secretly planned to throw herself under a train. Here death is viewed as a place where the self will survive in a state similar to that of a sleeping infant, perpetually united to her parental figures. To kill the body seemed to be the way of eliminating the obstacle to realizing this phantasy of fusion.

Phantasy of self-punishment: A ten-year-old anorectic girl dreamt she took her brother's motorbike, drove it over a cliff and died. This dream suggested that the girl was trying to 'act out' the idea of having to be punished for the incestuous relationship she had had with her grandfather. The experiences of speaking about her sexual experiences during the assessment had created a rupture in her obsessive control of the aggression of the severe superego and her masochism risked being 'acted out' through suicide.

Phantasy of revenge: Being brought by the parents to a doctor because of a severe difficulty in eating is often experienced by the child as a betrayal. The child feels that the parents are abandoning her to the persecutory presence of doctors who forcefully break her defences through feeding her. One child had repetitious dreams of world disasters including one in which an atom bomb dropped, killing everyone. This prepubertal child had concealed weights in her underclothes to make the doctors believe she was an acceptable weight. When the weights were discovered and she was no longer able to prevent her parents from bringing her to hospital, she slashed her wrists, jumped off the windowsill and tried to strangle herself. In this way she tried to attack the parents' loved child and also the parents for 'not loving her enough' to let her remain at home.

Phantasy of elimination: The body with its hunger for food can be experienced as a nuisance or as a threat to the omnipotent control of the anorectic part of the self. For this reason, the body, as a source of conflict to the fragile self, has to be eliminated. A 13-year-old told me during her assessment: 'At times I dream of saying goodbye to my classmates, then eating all I want and throwing myself into the pond. This dream makes me happy.' In this way the body, with all its hunger is thus killed. This phantasy of death contains the killing of the perpetual longing for her emotional and physical needs to be satisfied by the parents.

Claustrophobic phantasy: An emaciated child regularly dreamt of being in a lift with a group of good and bad people. Her good parents turned into horrible people and the bad people turned into terrible monsters. She was trapped inside the lift. Upon awakening she felt desperate.

All these dreams, containing a prevalence of psychotic anxieties, suggest that the child lacks a good internal figure who might protect her from her own destructive impulses. In such situations there is a strong risk of suicide. For this reason it is essential to establish, as soon as possible, a therapeutic relationship that helps the child to face her sense of desperation and supports her in avoiding her tendency to act out her destructive phantasies.

Psychotic thoughts associated with severe eating disorders

In the assessment process, the silence of a child affected by anorexia nervosa or pervasive retreat is often influenced by the presence of 'controlling voices', which impede speaking. A particularly anxious child who is talking without establishing a positive emotional link with the therapist may be obeying the orders of that which she herself defines as 'voices'. It is therefore important, for example, to invite the silent child to raise her hand if something in her thoughts orders her not to eat or threatens her when she speaks with the therapist. For some reason, the hands of the child are often freer than the mouth and are able to signal or play with dolls in a way that reveals aspects of the child's emotional life (Magagna, 1996).

Anna, a 14-year-old anorectic girl, seemed very anxious while speaking very quickly. I asked her if there were voices inside her head. Surprised by my question, she replied with relief,

> Yes, there are three furious voices who speak to me. They threaten me when I make a mistake or don't obey their orders. They prohibit me from eating certain things and they criticize me for not following a meticulous programme that involves starving myself.

After she disclosed their presence, 'the voices' criticized her for speaking to me. They were such forceful, cruel and demanding voices that she felt she had to kill herself because she felt unable to bear their loudness. When I asked why she had not spoken about them before, she replied, 'You hadn't asked. Also, I was afraid that you would think I was crazy.' Through Anna, I became aware of how important it is to ask the young person about 'voices', which may be linked with psychotic anxieties, instead of waiting for them to be spontaneously revealed.

External events which may accompany the onset of an eating disorder

Children with severe eating disorders generally do not possess a flexible internal structure that supports their more overwhelming feelings (Rey, 1994). For this reason they are dependent primarily on external figures and are easily overwhelmed by conflicts with the people around them. A large proportion of the children suffering from anorexia nervosa feel that the illness was triggered by external events. Many claim to have been teased by important people, for example their parents or close friends, who had made them aware of a tendency towards fatness. Other frequently cited precipitating events are a sense of deprivation or loss created through a change of school, the divorce of parents, the return of the mother to work after she has been primarily at home looking after the children and the father's loss of his job. In addition to these precipitating events, the first intimate sexual contact, followed by separation from a boyfriend or girlfriend can create, in someone excessively depending on friendships, a conflict so severe that eating feels impossible. Also, at least 25% of our inpatient children suffer from anorexia nervosa after having had what they experienced as a sexually abusive experience, even though it wouldn't necessarily be considered to be so by others. The excessive dependency on external figures must also be examined in the light of the type of relationship that the child establishes with parents, teachers and friends at school. The need to please teachers may demonstrate that high achievement is occurring in relation to an extremely critical superego which threatens abandonment or a sense of complete failure if one isn't at the top of the class. The necessity to win the favour of the teacher and to desperately cling onto scholastic success may mask persecutory fears deriving from a sense of internal damage connected with phantasies of aggressive competition to beat the others in the class by obtaining top marks.

Needing to be top of the class may also suggest a transference to the teacher, wishing 'to shine' in the teacher's eyes, representing the mother's gleam of appreciation of her child.

The family

Eating disorders have a complex origin. I find it useful to give each member of the family the possibility of speaking of his or her own experience of being in the family. It is important to explore the conflicts and any traumatic events within the family as well as looking at the family's resilience and emotional capacities. It is useful also to assess what capacities members of the family have to be aware of their feelings and to reflect upon them, to resolve conflicts and to demonstrate sufficient flexibility to permit both individuation and age-appropriate development of each child. It is also important to note what good parenting has been taking place prior to the onset of the eating disorder, in order to collaborate with the parents in caring for their child's physical and emotional needs. By the time the family arrives for a consultation, their healthier ways of being together have been disrupted by the child's anorexia nervosa symptomatology.

To do the assessment it is also necessary to have at least two family exploratory meetings to ascertain the role played by the anorectic child's behaviour in relation to the current family pattern of interaction. It is in fact possible that other family members, particularly the mother, can be utilizing anorectic symptoms for their own unconscious motives, thus making it more difficult for the child to make developmental changes. The family's atmosphere of suffering and conflict may be located in the anorectic child. The family interaction may include the parents' difficulties which include lacking the capacity to mediate conflict, bear mental pain and difficulties in creating a family and couple atmosphere of intimacy, trust and optimism.

After the family explorations it would be useful to ask what factors in the family pattern of interaction may contribute to or perpetuate the child's eating disorder and which are able by contrast to facilitate the healthy physical and emotional development of the family members. At times it is necessary for the child to be with foster parents who can provide a good transitional space before returning home from full-time hospitalization.

In assessing serious eating disturbances, it is of vital importance to ask about possible organic origins of the symptoms. In fact, the refusal of food, the loss of weight or inability to gain weight, vomiting attacks and depression are signs that also accompany serious organic pathology of a life-threatening nature. Also, even though consistent loss of weight is usually associated with anorexia nervosa, a disturbance of eating may develop in inflammatory bowel disease, diabetes, chronic infections, malabsorption syndromes, mesenteric artery syndrome, various kinds of cancer and brain tumours, which only gradually emerge. The doctor is not able to exclude the hypothesis of a disturbance of an organic origin through a physical examination alone and additional medical tests may be required. However, unnecessary medical examinations should be avoided when possible if the psychological criteria for anorexia nervosa are met (Lask, 1993).

Other medical aspects that one must keep firmly in mind are the physical consequences of starvation. Cardiac ventricle dysrhythmia, congestive heart failure, bradycardia and electro-cardiogram abnormalities are only some of the serious medical complications that accompany starvation. While dizziness syncope and hypothermia are present in 50% of the cases of anorexia nervosa, there are more rarely seen fatal complications such as oesophageal and gastric rupture or pancreatic problems. Death through anorexia nervosa most frequently occurs through complete lack of potassium, resulting in cardiac arrest. For this reason, it is absolutely crucial that the non-medical professionals, the family and the child herself are informed of this type of danger of death, which can be discovered through testing the blood for potassium levels. It is not appropriate to provide individual therapy without other external support that assists the child to eat. Furthermore, in the assessment period for a child who has lost weight or is vomiting, it is essential that the child is seen by a doctor who notes the weight in relation to height and age, and also the height in relation to age. If the family is not able to help the child to eat adequately and the physical state of the child is below 75–80% weight/height/age, weight recovery in hospital, or day-patient treatment involving helping the parents help the child to eat, is essential to avoid serious long-term complications. Nowadays, professionals talk about a normal BMI (body mass index) as being 16.3–24 for 15-year-olds and consider hospitalization when there is a BMI of 14 or 15 if the family is not able to help the child gain weight in the first few weeks after meeting the clinician.

Making a formulation of the problem and a treatment plan

Ideally, there should be a flexible approach to children with eating problems. The children who are referred a hospital eating disorder team, such as that in Great Ormond Street Hospital in London, are offered the following possibilities: immediate emergency hospitalization for approximately two weeks in a paediatric ward under the joint care of a paediatrician and psychiatrist; psychiatric hospitalization preferably in an eating disorder unit for young people; family therapy; or at least once weekly individual therapy alongside family therapy or work with parents on a weekly or fortnightly basis.

The need for hospitalization

If the family members are able to be involved in a therapeutic programme and in this way sustain the child in her physical and psychological treatment programme, then the child may remain at home. Admission to hospital is considered when the child does not have adequate emotional support in the home and/or is stuck in a sadomasochistic relationship with the parents who are not able to contain the anxiety generated by the child's eating disturbance or emotional conflicts. Lask (1993, p. 136) suggests that recovery in hospital, with the objective of augmenting weight gain by approximately 0.5 to 1 kg per week, should also be considered as a serious option if there are any of the following physical complications:

- weight loss such that the weight in relation to the child's height and age is less than 75–80% weight/height (14–15 BMI)
- dehydration
- poor circulation as suggested by low blood pressure, slow pulse and poor peripheral circulation
- persistent vomiting, which can lead to life-risking physical complications
- vomiting of blood, which may suggest a life-threatening tear in the oesophagus.

Likewise, children with a predisposition to suicide and those suffering from other accompanying psychiatric disturbances such as severe depression or psychosis may require hospitalization. If parents refuse treatment for a seriously ill child, it may be necessary to involve social workers to organize a meeting with the aim of providing adequate legal protection to ensure that the physical and emotional needs of the child are met.

Day treatment programme

The day treatment programme in our hospital includes a half day attendance for the family members for a period of approximately 12 weeks, which can be extended according to the needs of the family. This intervention programme is offered at the time of referral for treatment as well as following inpatient admission. The day programme includes the following weekly events: family therapy, individual therapy for the child with an eating disturbance, a parents' group, and a children's activity group. At times there is also a group for the siblings of the child with the eating disorder.

Outpatient programme

More than one anorectic child has expressed the fear: 'When I look all right on the outside, I am afraid no one will notice how bad I feel inside.' In saying this, she expressed her fear of having to continually display her 'starvation' for fear that others would do what she did, which was to ignore her inner emotional condition and focus only on weight gain and sexual development. In general, it is necessary to retain some form of treatment for at least a year, accompanied by follow-up appointments for at least 18 months. The length of treatment is necessary to help the child develop a more stable psychic structure. An 18-month follow-up has been shown to be helpful in preventing relapse.

Each of the various eating disorders are accompanied by disturbed psychic functioning, which includes denial of emotions. Such denial prevents taking care of the infantile part of the self and in this way interfere with the development of emotional maturity. For this reason, all the children presenting disturbances in eating are suitable candidates for individual psychotherapy. In practice, family therapy, because of its efficacy (Lock and Le Grange, 2015), is often offered without individual therapy because this is a limited resource within the national health service.

Even if family therapy is the treatment chosen, every child with an eating disorder is given several individual assessment sessions, separate from the family, in order that the child may think about her life, her feelings and difficulties that may later be addressed within the family therapy. As I approach an assessment interview, I bear in mind three young people, none of whom were initially disposed to discuss their difficulties in the family therapy. One is a 14-year-old anorectic girl who told me that she had never told the doctors, who had treated her for several years prior to seeing me, about repeated experiences of sexual abuse in her early childhood. When asked why not, she said, 'No one has ever asked about sexual abuse. I felt awkward in bringing it up myself. I was afraid my parents would blame me for the abuse having taken place.' The second young person told me she had never told anyone about 'her voices'. When asked why this was, she replied, 'I am afraid people would think I am crazy and anyway I like my voices for they keep me company and I am afraid of losing them.' The third young person, when asked about different suicidal impulses, said she had none. However, when I asked her to describe a dream, it conveyed such a picture of hopelessness and despair that I showed curiosity about what caused despair and then she answered, 'Well, I did secretly take an overdose of paracetamol but I don't want my mother to know.' Of course, it was important that I didn't let her leave the clinic until we thought together about how she might tell her parents right after the session and we thought further with her parents about her feelings and her safety.

The assessment phase is primarily designed to give the young person an opportunity to think about her life. This includes talking about her anorectic symptoms and her attitude towards her anorexia nervosa. Does she feel she has 'no problem' but that it is only her parents' problem or does she see the problems but doesn't really feel up to addressing them, or does she see that she has difficulties and have some motivation to begin to think about the developmental phase in which she is and the issues which create obstacles for her. It may be simply that the absence of a secure parent who will assist her in the task of mentalization is what has been present for quite some time. At other times it may be a crisis which cannot be discussed with anyone, because she trusts no one or doesn't even know how to put her emotional experience into words.

Beware of the 'intellectual mask' of the young person with anorexia nervosa or bulimia nervosa! An eating difficulty, whether it is bulimia or anorexia, involves the use of omnipotence and projection of feelings. Not telling the truth and concealing emotional difficulties is part of the weaponry of the anorectic defence and can be expected. For this reason the similar pattern of eating difficulties may mask a variety of psychiatric symptoms. A young person with an eating disorder may be experiencing vivid auditory or visual hallucinations or ever-present 'imaginary friends'. Because of the anorectic young person's use of primitive omnipotence to feel and appear 'normal', such pathological phenomena are frequently concealed.

In an attempt to gain a more in-depth understanding, it is important to provide an individual assessment of approximately an hour for each young person with an eating disorder. It is helpful to have at least one free-flowing assessment interview, in which the young person is encouraged to use the opportunity to tell the story of herself as she would like to tell it, rather than simply supply information. Factual information can be gained in a subsequent interview and in other therapeutic settings. In individual assessments I have sometimes found it helpful to ask the young person, particularly children, to draw a picture of a person. Then I ask the child to tell me about the person and create a story for that person. Subsequently, with the assistance of the child, I try to find similarities and differences between the person in the story and the child I am meeting. The rest of the session is used as a space for the child to explore dreams and other issues of her choice. Spontaneous play, discussion of dreams and drawings are also used for the younger child to elaborate upon conflictual emotional issues.

When a child or young person has difficulty in speaking about herself, I discuss her difficulty in meeting a stranger, her fear of my criticism and of me. I find it helpful to give her a family set of small cloth dolls and ask her to speak from the perspective of various family members, as I interview the doll family regarding 'their picture' of the young person's life in her family. I also encourage the young person to tell me a dream, any recurring dreams, and dreams from her past. In this way I gain access to the child's psychic structure. I try also to think about suicidal ideation and abuse with the child. I also begin by first asking, 'If in trouble, to whom would you turn?' I am very concerned when the young person says 'no one' or indicates only peers. I am aware this young person is unlikely to talk to me in an initial meeting about some serious problems, but if a very good emotional rapport is established, the young person is relieved to talk, for the first time, about some very serious emotional issues.

I am trying to discover the young person's internalized representations of the significant people in her life and their functions in relation to her. This is how I consider the child's psychic structure. The key components are a maternal figure, a paternal figure, sibling figures and the infantile self. These paternal and maternal figures are typically used by young people to represent the nurturing, protective, regulating and procreating roles of each parent, the grandparents, nannies and the roles of the siblings. It is important not to under-emphasize the supportive, destructive and problematic functions and roles of nannies and siblings (Magagna, 1996, 2005).

An examination of the maternal figure reveals the quality of nurturing and physical comfort and security provided, the capacity to receive distressed aspects of the infantile self and the ability to modify pain. Evaluation of the paternal figure includes noting the capacity to regulate emotion so that feelings are neither too intense nor too restricted, to differentiate good from bad, to provide limits and also a description of his moral code noticing whether or not rules are followed out of fear of punishment or out of concern for the well-being of oneself or others. An assessment of the nature of the relationship with siblings and peers includes looking at the way in which conflicts between love, jealousy, and anger are expressed in these relationships, and also noting the capacity to acknowledge the siblings' existence and needs. I often find that hostility of the child with an eating disorder towards the parents is displaced onto the siblings.

An assessment of the young person's relationship with other significant adults such as grandparents, teachers, relatives and nannies gives a fuller picture of the young person's attitudes towards authority, emotional support, separation and loss. My primary question during an assessment is: what capacity does the child have, in identification with internal figures, to compassionately understand her feelings and in that way to look after her own infantile self? In empathically listening to a child, I hear the child's stories and tone of voice, as well as noting my emotional and physical responses to the child's predominant attitudes to her experience.

I then develop a picture of world the young person, as a result of her experiences, has in her mind. These experiences will be the result of the interaction between her impulses, the phantasies arising from them and the external factors of her life, particularly the quality of the relationship with the primary attachment figures, generally the parents, and the quality of nurturing and understanding the young person has developed with these primary attachment figures. Evaluation of the child's relationship to the parents involves the place of emotional and intellectual nurture in the child's home life and her attitude to being taught and disciplined by parents and teachers. The nature of the relationship between the parents and the nature of their attitude to the young person must be considered. I also consider the child's capacity to allow the internal parental figures to be together in various creative ways, including procreation and the care of the siblings. This can be shown through scenes in dreams in which a couple are cooperatively doing something worthwhile.

The nature of the internal parental figures will be influenced not only by the qualities of real parents, but also by the child's own feelings towards them. A stable sexual identity is based upon acknowledgement of one's gender, as well as identifying with both internalized parental figures performing their task of looking after the infantile self and joining together in creative ways. The child's experience of her own body is influenced by these identifications and reflected in her sense of physical security and physical movement, as well as in the themes of her play, dreams, and stories. Lack of parental care as well as hostility to the parents can result in damaged internal parents and a lack of self-esteem as well as a lack of good feelings about one's body and sexual identity.

Later, always with the help of the child, I try to understand the similarities and differences between the person in the story and the child and the members in her family. The remaining time in the session is available to the child to explore her emotions as she wishes. I always ask specific questions about emotional and/or sexual abuse.

Rosa

I shall now discuss some material from two individual assessment meetings with a six-year-old girl who was having severe difficulties eating, resulting in her being considerably underweight. The family had already had some exploratory meetings and Rosa had undergone a comprehensive medical examination.

First session

Having long black hair and large dark brown eyes, Rosa, an attractive child of British-Filipino heritage, greeted me with a smile. On the table I had placed two sheets of drawing paper and a range of toys including animal and doll families. When she entered the room, I asked her to draw a person. Without hesitation she rapidly drew a woman with a wedding veil and said, 'It's a bride.' Above the bride she drew a bunk-bed with a squirrel on it, saying, 'The squirrel is going to sleep.' Across from the squirrel she quickly drew a heart-shaped sun with very sexualised lips. Subsequently she drew a man standing beside the bride.

Without my asking any questions, Rosa described how the man was not married to the woman, but they had two children, a boy of two years and a girl of seven. She added that the husband was working in the garden. When I asked about this, she answered, 'The wife is very angry with him because he hasn't bought her a wedding ring.' When I wondered why this was, Rosa complacently replied, 'The man was too poor. The wife sent him out to work because she is the boss in the house.'

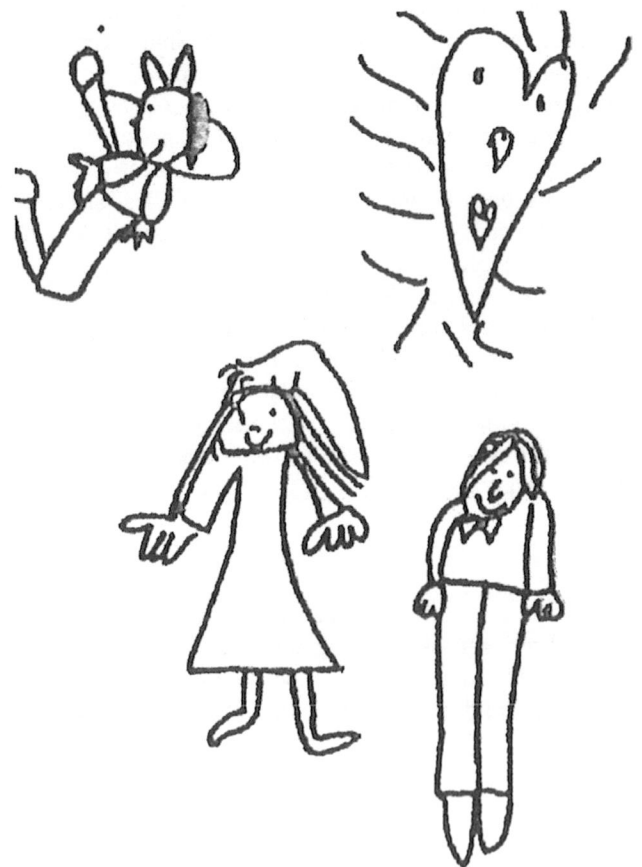

Figure 2.1 Man beside bride

As an afterthought, Rosa, spying a felt-tip pen, immediately exclaimed, 'Oh, how lovely, pink!' and drew another woman in very bright colours. Using scissors, she then cut out this mother and placed her on the white sheet alongside her three children, boys of four and two years and a girl of seven. On the same sheet were also drawings of other small children.

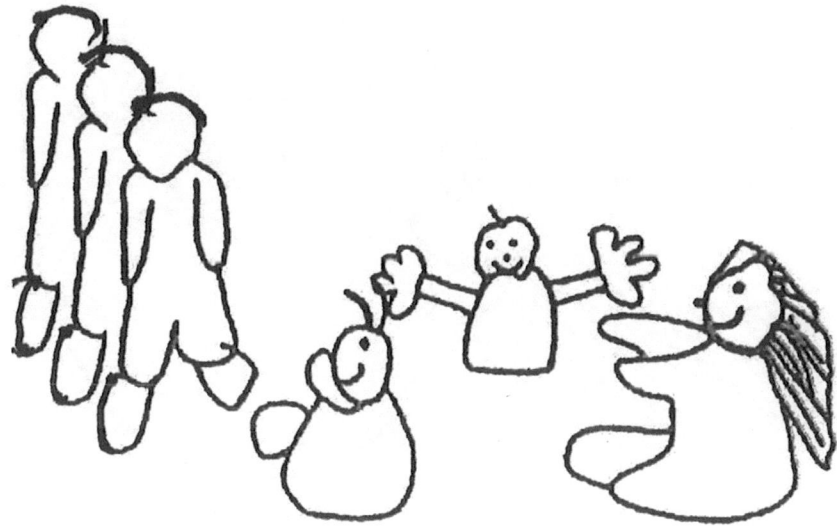

Figure 2.2 Mother with children

While describing these children, Rosa suddenly commented, 'At school the children hit and kick me.' Then, moving towards the divan, she leaned against it, moving her bottom up and down, as though she were mimicking an intercourse.

The next picture was of a tiny girl and a large man whom she said was the father. Drawing a circle around the two, she placed an enormous fish with an open teeth-lined mouth nearby.

She said, 'This big fish is going to eat the girl up and then it will eat up the father!' Then she made a mermaid with long blond hair. Accompanying this drawing was a short written sentence: 'I must save these two.' I asked Rosa, 'Why must the mermaid save the father and the girl. What is happening?' To this she replied, 'She must save the father and the little girl from getting eaten by the big fish.' I commented, 'Probably the girl is very frightened.' She nodded. I then asked, 'Are there any things which worry you?' She replied, 'I wish to be good. I want to eat my food and be healthy again.' I said, 'The little girl must be *very good*. Something makes her very frightened.' Rosa answered, 'The big fish,' and then repeated, 'The boys at school kick me and hurt me.' I suggested that we would need to think more about this with her parents.

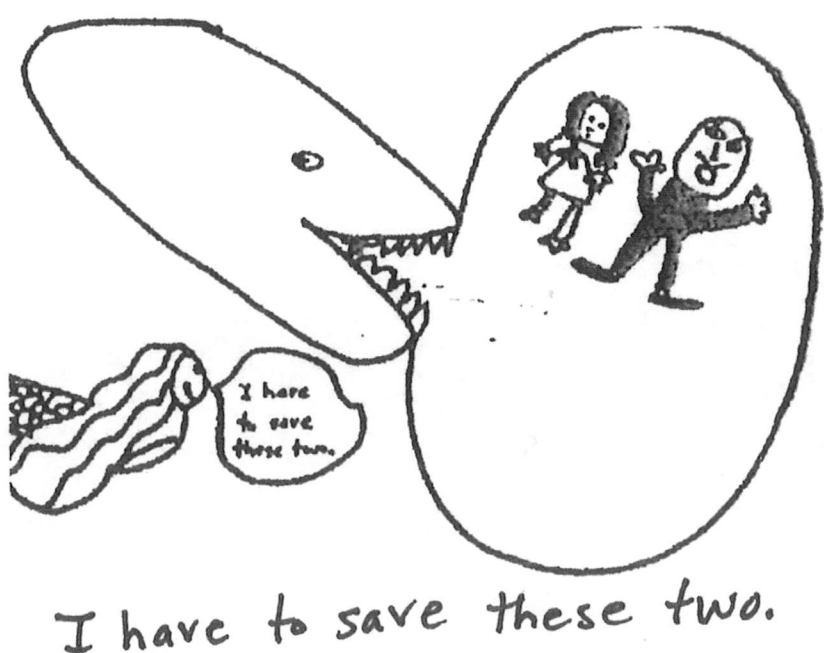

I have to save these two.

Figure 2.3 Frightening fish

Afterwards, when I told Rosa it was time to end our meeting, she didn't want to leave. Taking a piece of string, she tried to measure the end of the bulletin board. She wanted to know how long it was. Later, as we walked down the corridor, she kept looking at me. When we met her father, Rosa took my hand and did not want to let it go. Her father helped her put on her jacket and she then ran after me, looked directly at my face and puckered her lips in an attempt to kiss me goodbye.

Second session

When I saw her the following week, Rosa called me 'Mrs Gun'. Once inside the room she wanted to draw and amongst the many things she made was a little girl. Rosa explained, 'She has fallen into the water and is drowning.' She added:

> The swans have to help her. They are throwing out a rubber ring which floats toward her. This is a man with three, no four legs. He is trying to save her. The little girl in the drawing is saying 'ooh' to the man.

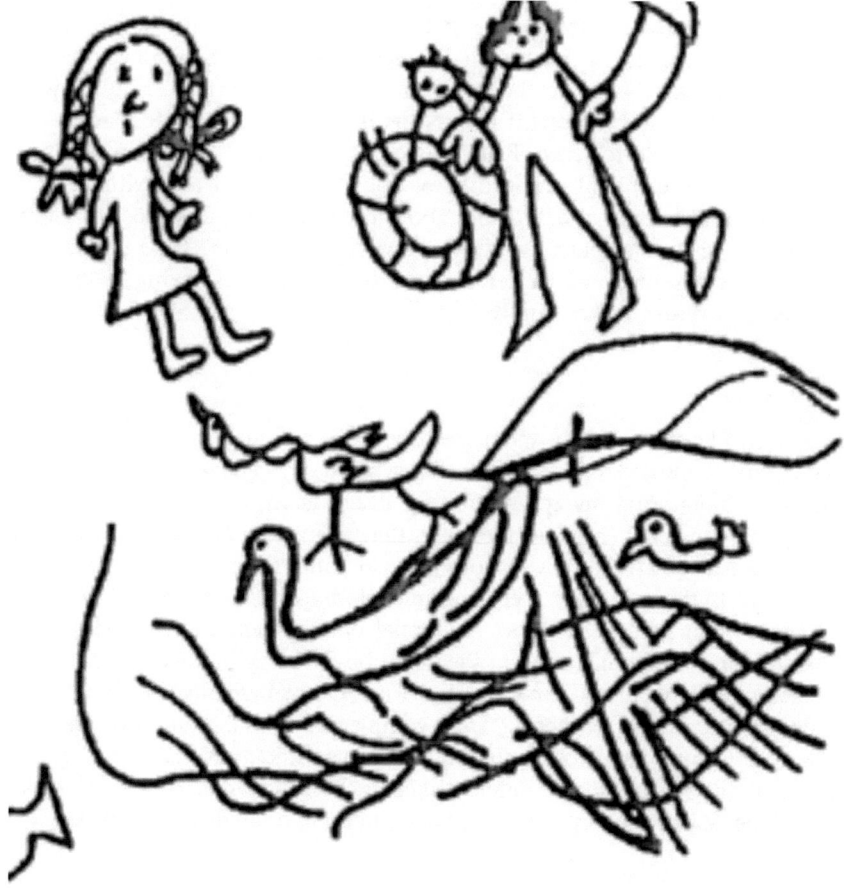

Figure 2.4 Drowning girl

While drawing the girl's open mouth, Rosa kept repeating the sound 'ooh', expressing differing strange feelings through her tone of voice.

Then, with a pencil, Rosa poked a white plastic horse. She then hurt my finger with her pencil, and laughed after I exclaimed, 'Ouch, you certainly want me to feel the hurt.' When I asked her what hurt her, Rosa answered that her mummy and daddy sometimes hit her. Her father hit her on the bottom. Pointing to her genital region, she said the children at school kicked her there. She added: 'But my mother kisses me on the bottom and sometimes says she will eat me up.'

Shortly afterwards, Rosa rested two cows on their sides and placed two calves in a position from which they could suckle from their mothers. She said that the calves were sucking for a long time and left them there for several minutes. Then there was a repetitious fight between the horse and the cow. Rosa described, 'In the end they killed each other.' She added that the elephant then came and ate the cow. Afterwards the baby doll lay in what Rosa called the 'daddy elephant's trunk' as if it had found a safe place.

When it was time to leave, Rosa was again desperate to remain with me. She grasped the elephant and the baby doll in one hand and with her free hand took hold of my hand. I talked about how she felt she needed to remain in a safe place to talk, play and show me what she felt. She tried to convince me to let her remain. I sensed her panic at the prospect of having to separate from me and return to her family.

Rosa's family

Since Rosa played and drew spontaneously during the assessment sessions, my interventions consisted principally in observing her, listening attentively to her words and monitoring my countertransference (Racker, 1974). I spoke only to amplify the significant emotions present at that moment in the session with Rosa. She was seen also in two family sessions with her parents and Datu, her three-year-old brother. In those sessions, there was an exploration of the family relationships and factors that influenced Rosa's emotional development and stunted growth. The question of what kind of harm she might be experiencing was also taken into consideration, both in the family sessions and more individual sessions. As is usually the case, Rosa's teachers had also completed a school profile regarding her.

I have tried to present Rosa's initial two sessions without excessive comment, in a way that allows clinicians of different theoretical inclinations to draw their own conclusions. My own interpretations of her internalized family are as follows.

The maternal figure

Two contrasting images of the maternal figure emerge. The image of the two calves sucking the teats of the cow suggests her wish for a prolonged experience of being mother's baby. There is some contemplation of the possibility of playing with mother as well as sharing her with others; however, the little brother, Datu, was initially left out of the drawing, suggesting some ambivalence about his arrival into her family. Separation from mother constitutes a problem for Rosa and she turns to her father as though she and he are the couple and mother is left out. The parental couple has been attacked and mother is attacked by jealous Rosa taking her place beside father. The imagined solution to Rosa's oedipal anxieties is to have the mermaid save the little girl and the man, representing father, from both being devoured by the big fish and drowning. The mermaid seems to represent an omnipotent structure to which Rosa returns in the absence of a containing internal mother. In the presence of a jealously attacked and then attacking and internal mother, the mermaid supports Rosa in the face of her overwhelming persecutory fears.

At the end of the sessions, Rosa clung to me desperately. It seems likely that when she does not succeed in maintaining a good external maternal figure or establishing a good internal supportive mother, in phantasy, Rosa resorts to biting mother. The maternal figure seems filled with Rosa's projections of destructive biting and assumes the shape of a terrifying fish threatening to devour the child.

These devouring and biting features emerge in Rosa's drawing of the large fish placed above the little girl. The devouring image is also implicit in her statement, 'My mother said that she is going to eat me up.' Mother may have said this affectionately, but Rosa had unconsciously perceived these words as a threatening response to her own ambivalent feelings towards mother which arose when she could not claim exclusive possession of her. One might also imagine that Rosa was in the grip of a devouring rage, perhaps linked to her experience during weaning or in conjunction with other separations from or lack of attunement with mother. It seemed that there was a persecutory mother-breast in her mind and this image was projected onto most food. Rosa may then have experienced most food as bad and unsafe to eat. Also, to avoid retaliatory biting attacks from the feared persecutory mother-breast, Rosa had to inhibit her own biting. She was having only soft foods: yoghurt without solid bits, milk, ice cream and creamy mashed potatoes.

Alongside the oral biting phantasies projected onto the mother are some sexual phantasies. When little Rosa is alone, like the squirrel in the bunk-bed intrusively watching the couple, she feels that she does not have a supportive internal figure, but only a sexual mother represented by the sun with sensual lips and by the bride who quarrels with her husband. Rosa's wish for union with either one of her parents implies that Rosa is a rival to both father and mother and thus the quarrelling couple may be linked with Rosa's own attack on the parental couple's union.

The paternal figure

Initially the paternal figure seems to be presented as a strong and protective figure that rescues the little girl. However, immediately afterwards Rosa draws a circle around the little girl and the father. This suggests some secret oedipal link, with the mother as a devouring and rivalrous figure. The paternal figure often reveals itself as weak, dominated by a maternal figure, more potent, angry and bossy, such as shown when the wife makes her husband work, while complaining that he does not provide a wedding ring and is poor.

The siblings and peers

Rosa portrays a scene in which she is able to share mother's nurturance with other siblings, but she did initially omit her three-year-old brother, Datu, from the drawing. Rosa's problem arises, in the absence of mother, when she does not succeed in maintaining a positive internal protective maternal image. This is shown in the story of being left in school with children who kick and hurt her.

Consciously Rosa strives to be a good little mother for Datu, her younger brother. Perhaps Rosa's unconscious aggressive feelings towards her brother leads her to feel the schoolboys, filled with her projected aggression, are persecutory figures. For whatever reason she seems to be a scapegoat who gets into sado-masochistic situations with the boys at school.

Concluding commentary

Six-year-old Rosa, with severe eating difficulties, is an extremely anxious girl. She seems identified with an omnipotent figure, a pseudo-mature part of herself, possibly represented by the mermaid, to protect her from persecutory fears. While feeling very grown up, she is continually haunted by fears associated with damaged internal objects: attacking boys, quarrelling parents. Her biting attacks on the parental couple have resulted in her feeling alone with the mental image of a biting mother, hitting father and a couple arguing with one another. How many of Rosa's phantasies represent external events will become clearer in the family assessments.

Using her pseudo-mature identity, Rosa tries to be a partner for her father, but this arouses her fear of a retaliatory mother. She needs to feel 'grown up' and to have control of situations, but at the same time she is identified with a hungry, dependent and frightened child. The refusal of food and her difficulties in learning seem associated with the pain of being a child, with repressed aggressive feelings projected upon the maternal figure, whom subsequently she can neither trust and or depend upon. Impediments to thinking, learning and eating are perhaps linked with the fear of frightening and bad experiences entering her.

When Rosa's individual assessment was reviewed in conjunction with the family assessments it was apparent that the parents had a very conflictual marriage. While in the family sessions Rosa complained of being 'dead inside' and 'numb'. Individual psychotherapy was proposed for Rosa alongside alternating family therapy and work with the parents alone.

Ongoing assessment of a pervasively retreating child

In contrast to my role in assessing anorectic young people and the children like Rosa who spontaneously offered thoughts and played and drew in the session, each year I also have the role of assessing several children suffering from what, in the absence of a more precise psychiatric diagnosis, is defined as a pervasive retreat from life, nowadays often referred to as PAWS: Pervasive Arousal Withdrawal Syndrome (Nunn et al., 2014). These are children who do not eat, drink, walk, speak or care for themselves in any way for a period which varies from several months to over a year. Obviously without medical intervention these children would be destined to die. In a state of helplessness, unable to change their situation, they use various psychological protections. These protections barricade their heart and their mind in the face of desires for security, intimacy and food that represents life itself. These processes involve the massive denial of reality, bodily constriction or erotization, primitive omniscience and omnipotence (Magagna, 1987).

The children have withdrawn from every social contact and have refused food in the course of diagnostic interventions in a paediatric unit. Because they do not speak, it was necessary to make an extended therapeutic assessment using detailed observations of the child. In these assessment sessions I search for a way of speaking with the child in a descriptive way, using furry animals, puppets and doll families to illustrate in various ways the story of 'the little one' who searches for protection by curling up and staying still. I accompany this narrative with observations of the child's nonverbal communications ... a movement away from me or towards me, or a glance showing an interest in what I am saying. I speak of the child's life on the psychiatric unit. While doing this I use the dolls to represent events, for example a meeting with the parents, the nurse or some other child. Gradually the child begins to put feelings into silent play with the dolls. Later the child often begins to give more definite facial or hand signals, draw, write a few words or speak (Magagna, 1996).

I will now illustrate my assessment and understanding of a child suffering from this syndrome involving a withdrawal from life.

Dorsey

Dorsey, an Afro-Caribbean girl aged 11, with long black curly hair, was hospitalized in a paediatric unit for three months with a history of ill health which started with a fall and cut hip, followed by complaints of sore and cracked lips, mouth ulcerations, listlessness, and refusal to eat or drink. She became increasingly withdrawn and eventually stopped walking, eating, drinking and speaking, making only high-pitched moans. The naso-gastric tube had been in place for the three months that she had completely rejected both food and drink.

When I met her she was in a wheelchair. Her body was completely curled up and her face was entirely covered by her hands, arms and long black curly hair. Her bodily gestures and facial expressions to convey her bodily sensations and emotional experiences seemed paralyzed (Brenman-Pick, 1985). She did not respond with either a sound or movement of her body to any comments or questions, or any touch by either the nurses or her parents. Dorsey seemed to be using massive denial to block knowledge of her own physical suffering and emotional and physical needs.

After about nine months, when Dorsey finally began to speak, she said with conviction that she didn't have a family and both in the past and present she had had no significant relationship with anyone outside the unit. She behaved as if her past scholastic success had never occurred.

The assessment of Dorsey, as with the other children whom I have seen presenting similar problems, was a continuous process. It was important to remember, together with Dorsey, that parts of her body were idealised as sources of permanent sensuous comfort. Everyone, including the family, the hospital staff and myself, had become identified in her mind with her destructive impulses. The approach of people threatened Dorsey's primitive omnipotent protective structure leading her to feel terrified even when someone looked at her.

As a result, I felt it was important to avoid looking or talking too directly to her. She listened to me while I spoke of a child's search for safety, holding, as the subject, a toy animal or doll that tried in various way to find a secure place in its relationships with nature and animate figures. Dramatic enactments of the stories of the animals and dolls were not presented in front of Dorsey, but to one side. This enabled her to feel free to turn towards me without being constrained by a personal encounter that was still too threatening. The non-stop sameness of Dorsey's bodily sensations while she was curled up behind her hands often seemed more preferable to her than any emotionally significant understanding.

Gradually she began to peek through her hands or hair and with a quick turn of her head she glanced at the story represented by the animals and dolls. When she did this, I responded by acknowledging the possibility of her taking an interest in what was being said. Dorsey's hunger for life was stimulated by my following her reactions attentively and giving them emotional significance through the stories dramatized beside her.

The stories initially revolved around the theme of massive denial of reality, bodily constriction, eroticization and primitive omniscience and omnipotence. Here are some examples of how I followed Dorsey's nonverbal responses and shared some of my understanding with her, using third person narratives rather than talking to her directly saying 'you feel'. I spoke in third person for it seemed less threatening to her. Also I felt she was able to reach towards what I was saying, rather than having the experience that my understanding was being intrusively directed towards her. The following are some examples of my speaking to her:

Massive denial: Dorsey was completely hidden behind her hands, arms and long curly black hair. Holding a doll in a curled up position, I said, 'It is terrible. What shall I do? I must hide away from everything. I shut my eyes. I close my mind. I must keep away from everyone to feel safe.'

Bodily constriction and erotization: Dorsey pressed her hands tightly against her face and her body was completely curled up into a ball shape. Using a doll in a curled up position I said,

> I don't like being here. This doesn't feel nice. It is frightening, but my hands are good, they comfort me. I can hold onto them. What I have to comfort myself is good. What comes from the Jeanne is frightening.

Mummy comes and then mummy walks away. Then I remain in a very unsafe place. I don't like being away from mummy.

Primitive omniscience and omnipotence: Dorsey secretly observed me and the room when I was not looking directly at her. I held the doll to say,

> I can notice what is going on. I need to notice every little change to avoid danger. I need to know. I can only trust what comes from me. I can only rely on what I can do for myself. I can take care of myself. I must hide myself, protect myself from everyone. I must watch everything that is happening to make sure that I am safe.

My impression is that the only way in which a child like Dorsey can be helped to abandon her attachment to self-limiting protections measures is through a relationship with a trustworthy person who responds attentively as a mother would be to a frightened baby who feels helpless (Magagna, 2002). These modes of providing understanding of very primitive emotional experiences and body sensations seem appropriate during various phases of development of a child pervasively retreating from life.

Initially it seems important to interpret the child's need for a secure place and a way of holding herself safely together. When the child used the 'blockading thumb' of protective measures, I interpreted her feeling of being safely away from danger, using her body, her hands, her curled up position to make herself feel better. It was significant to note that the child felt that using her body to separate herself from others felt good, while the external world felt terrifying and bad. Later it was important to verbalize a deeper understanding of the significance of the child's movements, while positioning myself at her side and dramatizing a story around her current emotional preoccupations and the events occurring around her. It was useful to provide a concrete focus of attention for the child using the third person of the character in the story in progressive stages of emotional intensity, moving from using objects such as building blocks, then toys, then animals and later the human doll family.

Development of an attachment to the key therapeutic care workers

Gradually Dorsey looked more directly at her primary workers and wanted them to notice her. Initially we described her feelings of panic or rage about our misunderstanding her and our not meeting her wishes or needs. On the occasions in which we succeeded in enlightening, interesting, nurturing and showing understanding of her present emotional wishes and needs, Dorsey turned to us like a sunflower turning to the sun. Gradually she became capable of taking in our understanding and then discovered the possibility of growing psychologically. (After one year of inpatient treatment, Dorsey was eating well, walking, living normally, expressing her feelings verbally, integrating well with friends and working successfully in school.)

My impression is that the only way in which a child like Dorsey can be helped to abandon her attachment to self-limiting protective measures is through a relationship with someone who responds attentively as a mother would respond to a frightened baby (Magagna, 2002). These special modes of providing understanding of very primitive emotional experiences and body sensations were appropriate during the various phases of development of a child experiencing a pervasive retreat from life.

Initially it seems important to interpret the child's need for a secure place and a way of holding herself safely together. When the child used the 'blockading thumb' of protective measures, I interpreted her feeling of being safely away from danger, using her body, her hair, her curled up position to make herself feel better. It was significant to note that the child felt using her body to separate herself from others felt good, while the external world felt terrifying and bad. Later it was important to verbalize a deeper understanding of the significance of the child's movements while positioning myself at her side and dramatizing in a story around her current emotional preoccupations and the events occurring around her.

It was useful to provide a concrete focus of attention for the child using the third person of the character in the story in progressive stages of emotional intensity, moving from using objects such as building blocks, then toys then animals and then later the human doll family. Gradually it was possible to note the emergence of moments of interest and attachment to the therapist. In particular it was possible to note when the child felt the therapist was a good figure and to understand and permit the development of an intense dependency. Subsequently interpretations focused in more detail on the way in which the therapist was experienced by the child. The therapist could be felt as non-understanding, irritating because late or absent, speaking too much or being too silent. Later interpretations revolved around the therapist as a source of jealousy because of her speaking to or looking at others.

After sufficient working on the therapist as a focus of attention, the therapist was subsequently described as a person able to feel projections from the child such as the feeling of being abandoned or no good. When there was a sense that the feelings projected into the therapist could be contained sufficiently within the child, the child was helped to explore and express feelings of panic, hurt and rage regarding not being understood and not having her therapist and primarily workers meet her needs.

If the feelings of the child were too intense and/or conflictual, I dramatized the conflict using the dolls, representing the child who spoke with me, the child who cried when I was unable to understand her or went away from her. At times I spoke as though I were the child, identifying with what I imagined the child felt and using the child's tone of voice. Later, through speaking on behalf of the child, I would suggest that maybe the child was feeling as I had suggested.

My experience is that, if the external figure furnishes an experience containing vitality, interest, and nurturance relevant to the actual emotional life of the child, the child begins to turn towards the therapist. A dependency on the therapist's understanding is thus created. There is a gradual diminishing reliance on the child's primitive omnipotent measures to protect herself and subsequently the child begins to trust the therapist, workers and parents: in this way introjection of good internal parents is possible and the psychological growth of the child proceeds.

Conclusion

I have endeavoured to show how important it is to take into consideration the way in which one can therapeutically communicate with very distressed children. Every human activity has an intrinsic emotional significance. One of the most important needs of a human is to be profoundly understood in an intimate relationship with another human being. For these reasons, I firmly believe that no child, whether or not she is in a non-speaking and/or emaciated state, should be deprived of an opportunity for therapeutic understanding.

I do not share the view that individual assessments and psychotherapy are solely for the child who is fundamentally healthy, intelligent and able to be articulate about emotional experiences. However, to work safely with such ill children, it essential to assess the physical and emotional strength of the treatment setting and the physical health of the eating disordered child. It is of the utmost importance for the psychotherapist to determine what intensity of contact is tolerable to a child and to modify the approach accordingly. It is also important to realize that the assessment process needs to involve observing and describing nonverbal communication rather than simply trying to get verbal communication from children who initially may not be able to put their emotional experiences into words.

Chapter 3

Individual psychotherapy in the context of a multidisciplinary eating disorder team

All repressed feelings accumulate inside and become more and more threaten-ing as time goes on. The error is to ignore them. They may be huge, blood-thirsty, and glow in the dark ... they lose their power as soon as they have been ... painted, danced, sung, or spoken.

(Cameron 1996, p. 14)

Introduction

Marie, a 12-year-old with anorexia nervosa, was asked in her individual assessment why she felt no one liked her. She answered: 'Because I'm fat.' 'Would you like to draw a picture of yourself?' I asked. Marie hesitated for a moment and then drew the picture shown in Figure 3.1.

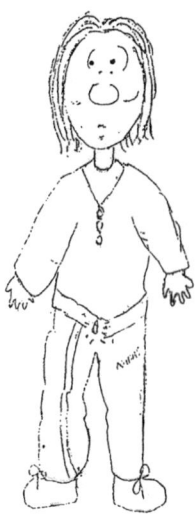

Figure 3.1 Marie's self-portrait

DOI: 10.4324/9781003044970-4

'Yes, you feel very fat indeed,' I said. 'I am very fat,' she replied. And now how do I respond, I thought? Despite her experience of being fat, Marie is outwardly very thin and emaciated. No matter how often people tell her she is thin and not fat, her reality is that she is unlikeable because of 'fat'.

In the first instance the focus of psychodynamic therapy is to accept Marie's physical and emotional experiences and to help her develop a capacity to think about them. Firstly, she needs to hear that I empathize with her and that I wish to understand the nature of her experience of feeling unliked and unlikeable. Marie also needs to understand that I accept her feeling that she is obviously filled with something disgusting, something that makes her bloated with this terrible substance she calls 'fat'. I cannot move forward therapeutically until Marie feels that I accept her physical experience of fatness as well as her emotional experience of being disliked. Saying that I feel she is thin, not fat; is attractive, not unattractive; is likeable, not unlikeable, would be rejecting Marie's painful inner reality.

Psychodynamic psychotherapy involves listening while constantly being physically and psychologically attuned to everything that is being experienced within the young person and the therapist. A psychotherapeutic exploration filled with a wish to know and a capacity to endure confusion and not knowing Marie's inner reality is important for her. In the first meetings with an anorectic young person I experience a kind of emotional barricade of varying degrees when I offer understanding. I imagine that this barricade has been erected as the young person's way of feeling 'held together' and secure in the absence of an inner psychic structure capable of mentalization alongside my thinking with her. An inner psychic structure capable of mentalization gives meaning to emotional experiences and puts them into some manageable psychological form. The task of psychoanalytic psychotherapy is to help Marie to develop this capacity for mentalization. Marie's 'barricading omnipotent self' seems to consist of obsessional control, an intellectual detachment from emotional experiences, denial of a more complex emotional life and non-stop forms of exercise such as running and swimming. The omnipotent self is against depending on others who are feared to be unable or unwilling to meets one's emotional needs. Some severely anxious young people, fearing disintegration, hold onto the omnipotent self for dear life. Over time the omnipotent self becomes a part of the personality structure fulfilling the following functions:

- It attacks the strength, goodness and vitality present in the emotional link with the therapist.
- It attacks the mutual understanding which is being created with the therapist.
- It attacks the 'self' in the young person trying to get in touch with feelings.

- It attacks the link with life by promoting the symptom of not eating.
- It uses obsessional control rather than depending on the primary caregivers or therapist.

Initially, the omnipotent self was felt to be so destructive that Marie said, 'I just want to die.' 'Let me die.' 'There is no point in living.' 'If you love me, you will let me die.' She covered her face with her hands and hair and tried to keep out of the world of people who had turned into enemies and persecuting intruders. This feeling of the world turning bad had been exacerbated by the rows with her parents who had attempted to make her eat, so that she wouldn't starve to death, and by the fury with her parents for admitting her to hospital. On the surface of herself, Marie experienced this hospital admission as implying that her parents didn't love her, but rather just wanted to abandon her to other caregivers. Only later was she able to accept that her parents had saved her life through the admission to hospital.

Much time in the initial meetings with Marie was spent with her not speaking, with her head down, while I talked about what I felt her experience might be. My description included a story of her feeling she had to close her mind, close her mouth, close off her contact with her parents and others. I said that somehow she felt she had to close herself off from everyone and everything including food and television.

I told Marie that what was complicated for her was that it was her parents who had decided that she needed hospital admission, which included having psychotherapy. I accepted her feeling that coming into the therapy room, therefore, could initially feel like being force-fed. For this reason, I felt it was essential to point out that, whereas Marie may not have had a choice about coming to therapy, she did have a choice about whether she spoke or did any work in the therapy through thinking alongside me. I said she could think or not think when she was silent with me. She was free to use her capacities. No one could make her think!

At the same time, I was aware that many of Marie's sensations, emotions, and perceptions had not yet been put into symbols suitable for her to think about them. They were not encapsulated in words: they were only located in her body. For this reason the sessions involved my using my counter-transference experiences to inform the way in which I described to Marie emotional experiences we shared in the room. I avoided asking many questions when it was clear she would not answer them. Instead I just reviewed her life and discussed our experiences in the room. At times, when Marie felt very withdrawn into herself, I tried to avoid being intrusive by having dialogues with myself while my eyes focused to the side of her as I told stories using puppets, dolls and stuffed animals. I implied that when she felt so inclined Marie could chose to turn to my understanding or if she felt my understanding was too intrusive, she was free to shut her eyes, cover her ears and turn away from me.

It is striking how often an older adolescent may take an interest in these 'children's things' as a means of enacting some as yet unformed verbal thought. It may be simply the force or gentleness of a gesture in handling the toys that conveys a sense of persecution, hurt, or anger. For example, in one therapy session a 12-year-old boy, with selective eating, said, 'I'll never play with those toys. They are for younger children.' However, he frequently began sessions by rolling a train over the body of several dolls' bodies or knocking the dolls' heads together. As is often the case, his hands were able 'to speak' first. They led the way for me to explore how going to sleep was difficult for him, because at night he was continually haunted by nightmarish creatures in his dreams, which he had kept private throughout much of his life. Attacks on important people in his life had damaged them and turned them into night monsters which in the day were projected into many foods he considered 'bad'.

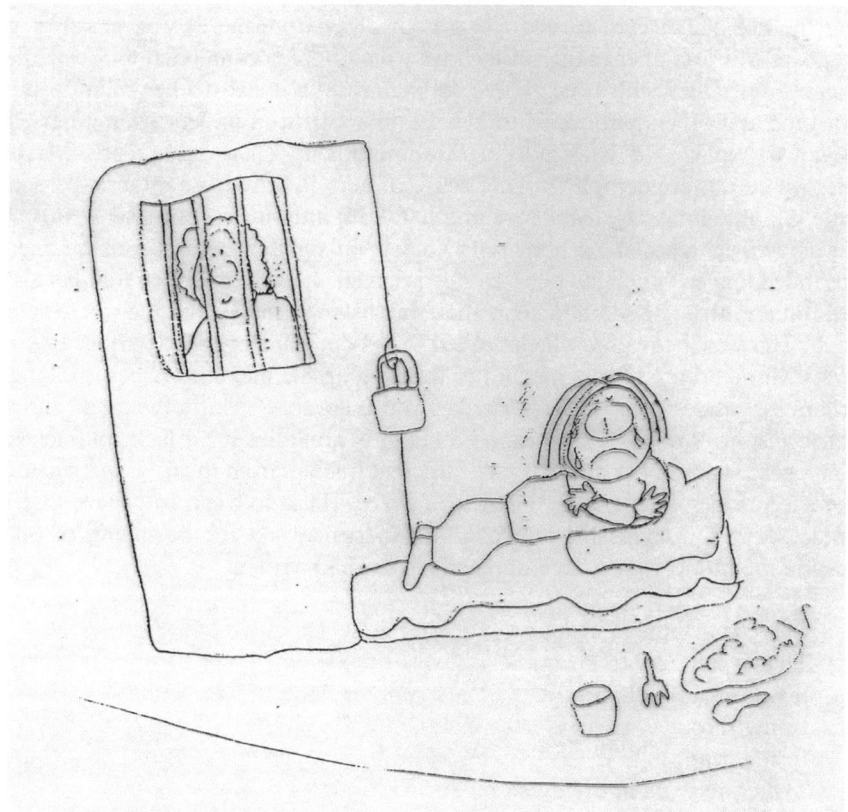

Figure 3.2 Drawing of a girl barricaded in a prison cell

As therapy progressed, Marie illustrated her important dilemma through a drawing in which a locked door imprisons her and also barricades her against a relationship with her mother (Figure 3.2). Marie's arms are used to comfort herself and also to control herself so she does not eat the food on her plate. In the drawing she lets me know she is crying, but not yet able to turn to her mother, father or me. The anorectic child is basically unable to achieve dependency in an intimate relationship. She has experienced disappointment, hurt and/or trauma. From an early developmental phase in her life she fears unreliability of people upon whom she might depend and has become insecurely attached to important caregivers. As a result she feels she can only count upon herself and her own means of control by the omnipotent self to cope (Rosenfeld, 1987a). This barricade of the omnipotent self leaves an inner self starved of understanding and support. For example, suicidal impulses or even suicidal attempts can be hidden from the parents in alliance with this controlling omnipotent self.

Gradually in psychotherapy, through her bodily and vocal gestures including the use of her eyes turned towards or away from me, it was possible to discover Marie's inner reality of feelings which have accumulated and become bigger and uglier with time. These feelings can be linked to her relationship with me and others important to her. In time a path of understanding herself began to replace the barricade of the omnipotent self. Consequently Marie discovered a more complex, richer sense of herself with more intense, passionate infantile longings, fears, love and hate. But although Marie's sense of self developed, her sense of her body-self as being 'fat and ugly' was fully maintained for much longer. Much later she revealed that she had voices which told her she was fat and that she shouldn't eat, shouldn't listen to me ... and they were very loud! This was her reality, which needed to be deeply understood (Farrell, 1995).

As Marie began to trust me and to think alongside me, I asked her, 'Tell me, what else besides your "fatness" makes you unlovable?' Marie then gave me a fuller answer: 'I'm shy, quiet, scared other girls won't like me. I lack confidence. I'm less clever than the others. I have different hobbies from them.' Experiencing my acceptance of her bodily 'ugliness' enabled Marie to begin to believe that I could tolerate disagreeable and painful experiences. At the beginning of one session she brought me a note upon which she had written:

> There is a sadness inside
> That is not able to go out.
> It makes me feel bad
> In my throat
> In my head
> There are tears in my eyes
> Crying in my voice
> Creating confusion in my heart.
> But slowly

The cry inside me
Becomes a scream which comes out.

I pondered to myself, 'Why did she need to write a note?' As I saw her looking at my face I realized she was wondering if I would be sufficiently responsive to her before she dared to further explore of her emotional experiences.
Schore (2002) states that in order transform the patient's distress, the therapist
must 'go beyond mirroring'. More than the clinician's verbalizations, it is his
nonverbal activity – the physical containment by the therapist of the patient's
disavowed experience – that needs to precede verbal processing (Dosamantes,
2002, p. 362). I remembered that, during her infancy, Marie had had a
depressed mother who, as a result, was probably not so able to be so responsive and mindful of her new baby. In receiving her note, I felt I concretely had
to hold Marie's crying 'baby-self' thrust into my hands and heart. I had to
show her that I had sufficient strength and hopefulness to accept her sadness,
her crying and her protesting screams.

Basic principles of psychodynamic psychotherapy

Providing a reliable setting and working on separation issues

Now that Marie was more fully conscious of her vulnerable 'baby-self' she
began to experience again some of the early anxieties of infancy which had
been hidden by her omnipotent self from both her and her mother. It is for
this reason that all the basic ingredients of a good relationship had to be
present in my therapeutic relationship with Marie. Firstly, I needed to be
prompt and reliable in the provision of therapy sessions so that Marie would
know that there was a regular, predictable rhythm to our being together. At a
minimum, weekly intervals provided an opportunity to build trust in a therapeutic relationship. I had in mind that therapy should be consistently at the
same time, the same place, with regular predictable breaks, announced well in
advance. I was clear that sufficient working through of Marie's attachment to
me and the therapy, as well as her feelings about separation from me and the
therapy, need to be considered before the break.

Following the break, the way in which Marie had experienced the separation, and how she experienced me after the break, required full consideration.
The implications of Dr John Bowlby's (1969, 1973, 1980) work describing
attachment, loss and separation need to be fully understood by me when
working therapeutically with Marie's very vulnerable 'baby-self'. Her 'baby-
self' was having another opportunity to be born, to be known and to develop
through being sensitively accepted, attended to and thought about in the
therapeutic encounter. I realized that until Marie had an attachment to her
work with me, a break from therapy was a relief. However, once Marie
became more positively responsive to our jointly developing understanding of

her, she was sometimes distressed by endings of sessions, breaks between the sessions and holidays and ruptures in my attunement to her. When Marie felt angry and/or abandoned by me she sometimes returned to the omnipotent self which promotes starving and exercise to 'hold the self together' emotionally. After a two-week break, Marie would sometimes avoid eye contact and be detached emotionally from me. It would take some time to re-discover a warm, more open relationship with each other.

Detachment could occur through Marie denying her dependence on me, saying, 'therapy isn't important anyway'. At times, detachment also occurred because Marie experienced a painful sense of loss of the therapy, rage and anger towards me for leaving her. Her hostility turned both me and her food into receptacles for her hostility and were then experienced concretely as 'not good'. Similarly, Marie's body, filled with her anger and this image of me as a 'not good therapist' was sometimes experienced as ugly and fat and she began to lose weight to get rid of the bad feelings. I also have to admit that sometimes after a holiday it was difficult for me to immediately locate myself in a good position in relation to Marie. This was particularly difficult when she had lost contact with all the work which we had done together before the break. It was painful for me to be rejected by her and I had to work through meaning of her evocation of my feelings of being unimportant.

As well as providing a trustworthy, reliable therapeutic encounter, an empathic listening and thinking space for the Marie and for my own countertransference feelings was essential.

The gradual unfolding of the infantile self versus use of the omnipotent self

Marie arrived for treatment having suffered from anorexia nervosa for eight months, during which time she had had an unsuccessful hospital admission. She had an early childhood history of obsessional behaviour dating from around age five. This seemed linked to the arrival of a baby sister that promoted extreme jealousy and hatred, which she attempted to control through obsessional rituals. In the absence of an inner psychic structure 'to hold herself together' (Bick, 1968), the obsessional rituals were also used to deal with all sorts of intense destructive, needy and loving feelings. When distressed, Marie retreated to her bedroom and listened to some voices dictating that she should walk back and forth from one wall to the other. At school she performed well academically and become excellent in gymnastics. The main problem, as she perceived it, was that she was superficially liked, but had no real friends. At 12, when she arrived for therapy with me, Marie complained that she was being teased at school. Her parents were also experiencing serious marital conflict accompanied by denial of conflictual difficulties both for themselves and the children.

Through my providing a regular, frequent and consistently timed therapy sessions as well as a listening and thinking place in my heart, Marie slowly found that the closed 'protective door' to her inner experiences opened so that she could slowly share as much as she was capable of feeling at one time. In the presence of my empathic listening, her intellectualized phrases began to be characterized by a connection to her deeper emotional experiences. Marie subsequently began to experience relief and even take pleasure in knowing herself more fully and understanding what was contributing to her anorectic symptomatology. The unfolding process of the infantile self in the therapy was primarily led by Marie, using the more mature part of herself to think alongside me. As a psychodynamic therapist I could give depth of meaning to her words, thus holding her emotionally so she could tolerate some of the pain, joy and relief in getting to know more about herself and the nature of her relationships with significant others. Marie's journey was one in which she was free to explore as much or as little of herself as she felt able and willing to get to know.

My stance, involving the 'mentalization process' (Fonagy et al., 2004), was to continually think about our experience of talking together and make interpretative open questions to encourage Marie to begin thinking about her experiences. Here is an example of some of the questions going on in my mind:

- What is happening now?
- Why is Marie saying this now?
- Why is Marie behaving like this?
- Why am I feeling as I do now?
- What has happened recently in the therapy (or with the hospital community or family) to justify this?

I realize that Marie creates anxiety in me in an attempt to rid herself of the mental pain she is feeling. I talked about her feeling that I needed to be in perfect harmony with her point of view and her hostility to me if I wasn't agreeing exactly with her. She said she didn't speak with her family because no one in the family liked her. I said, 'It might be to do with your hate and anger too when they don't do let you do exactly what you want to do.' She said, 'I won't come to therapy anymore if you speak like that ... and I'll stop eating too!'

Her 'protective door', which I call her omnipotent self, using obsessional and anorectic symptomatology, had often served as her method of preventing being flooded by too much psychic pain, too much intense pleasurable emotion or too many bodily sensations. The omnipotent self is felt to be superior to the adults, to be independent of human bodily and emotional needs, and to be in control. Marie was attached to her omnipotent self, her 'brick wall' as she called it, rather than being able to depend on others. 'Anorexia is my best friend. It is always with me,' Marie says. 'I don't want to lose that!' Her omnipotent self had dominated Marie's healthy infantile self and thus it had been hidden from both herself and her caregivers. It was noticeable how when we discussed emotional experiences which were too painful, Marie would turn to her omnipotent self and there would then be a discourse on calories, weight, fatness. Thinking about the emotional point of our previous discussion was then temporarily obliterated until I returned to it.

The development of a dependent, trusting relationship with me and a sufficiently secure and containing external environment to allow Marie to 'open the door' to her suffering took time. On the other hand, helping Marie restore her physical health through weight gain needed to occur at about 0.3 to 0.5 kg per week. Because of medical complications associated with emaciation, Marie's weight needed to be restored in a far shorter time than the time required for her emotional self to be sufficiently healed. It was important for me to remember that adequate weight restoration did not mean that she was psychologically healthy, it just meant that her body was not suffering.

Transference and countertransference

> ...save me from the thoughts men think
>
> In the marrow bone;
>
> He that sings a lasting song
>
> Thinks in the marrow bone.
> ('A Prayer for Old Age', W. B. Yeats, 2001)

Communication is always taking place in therapy. It is a luxury for the therapist to have communication through words from the young person. However, much of what needed to be understood was first put into words and given meaning through my physical and emotional experiences felt when anticipating Marie's arrival for therapy, or my sitting in the therapy room with Marie, my pausing to think of my experiences after Marie had left the session. This acknowledgement of my own emotional experiences is what comprises my 'countertransference'. My countertransference experiences, forming my intuition, represent the primary fulcrum for making a timely interpretation, sensitively attuned to Marie's current emotional experience and her capacity to tolerate mental pain and the pleasure of emotional intimacy.

Transference and countertransference represent two components mutually giving life to each other and creating the relationship between the child and her therapist. Marie's therapy demonstrates this clearly. I shall be giving full illustrations of the therapeutic process later, but for the moment I would like to discuss these two concepts of transference and countertransference in a little more detail.

Marie's 'transference' to me is represented in all her communications and experiences in relation to me and the therapy. I assume that Marie transfers both positive and negative aspects of her parental figures – both internal and external – onto my personality which she experiences in working with me.

The nature of this transference then determines how Marie relates to me at any moment in time. 'Gathering the transference' implies scanning for unconscious infantile elements present in all the comments and stories Marie brings about experiences both outside the therapy and in her dreams. Simultaneously I am focusing on Marie's emotions that are most immediate and pressing as she talks with me or remains in silence, communicating non-verbally through her gestures.

Psychoanalytic psychotherapy is still often misunderstood as focusing on reconstruction of historical events, rather than dealing with the child's experience 'in the here and now' in the session. However, the primary tenet of current psychoanalytic thinking is that internal psychological change can best be facilitated through interpretations that meet anxiety and emotions at that present moment at which they are being experienced in the session. The material that Marie brought involved consideration not only of the content and mood of her communications. I also needed to consider precisely how the process of her bringing experiences, her tone of voice, her warmth or coldness, her emotional contact with the verbal content, provided clues as to what was happening between us in the session. Marie's remarks were also given meaning through their chronological sequence in the session. Often reading notes of Marie's session from the end of the session and then working upwards to the beginning of the session enabled me to understand more deeply Marie's transference anxieties in relation me in the beginning of the session. I also attempted to ask myself, 'What does this story about the past or the future, this story about something outside the therapy room, tell me about the unconscious nature of Marie's current preoccupations in relation to her therapeutic relationship with me?'

It was mainly through my countertransference that I felt and could understand what Marie felt about thinking with me in therapy. Often young people with eating disorders cannot find or will not share words with their therapist. Marie was no different. At times in the silence I would feel frustrated and impotent. This was particularly true when I was having difficulty attuning to my countertransference. But what is the countertransference really? It consists of various levels of emotional experience. First, countertransference is based on a connection with the child's impulses of love and hate and defences such as denial and projection. Secondly, countertransference implies receiving communications, which I am made to feel through Marie's enactments in the session. So, in this way, through identifying with Marie's internalized parental figures, I get hold of what her experience is of supportive or unsupportive internal parents and external parents. So, for example, at times I feel myself to be the useful parent; at times I feel myself to be the useless, ineffective parent; at times, I feel myself to be the intrusive or angry parent. At other times, for example, initially Marie was frequently late and I was to feel the waiting child, the unwanted child, the abandoned child, the angry child. Her enactments made me experience her projected unconscious feelings, which she could not bear to acknowledge in herself.

As well as this, Marie's transference to me is a response to my real and phantasized countertransference (Racker, 1974, p. 131). At different times Marie evoked problematic aspects of my personality by doing something angry provoking like talk with great pleasure and a smile on her face about doing 100 push-ups, knowing that I would find it absurd, and anger provoking to discover that she was exercising so strenuously at such a low weight. Her unconscious had a talent for seeking out and projecting into the more fragile, problematic aspects of my personality. Marie could project into my wish to be all-knowing, or my wish to be a mother, or she could evoke aggression in me and at times I would be denying my own hostility (Brenman-Pick, 1985). In particular, Marie often projected into my guilt about not being a loving or adequate person in some way. If I, as a therapist, could be still and in the silence listen to what was going on deeply within myself in the presence of Marie, then there was no need for me to question her penetratingly in order to extract some words from her.

Problems in making progress in therapy are often viewed by a therapist as the young person's difficulties. I know from my experience with Marie that some of the lack of progress was connected to my defending myself with intel-lectualization. When this splitting occurs in my own personality, Marie moves to a more superficial level within herself. Marie wouldn't be coming to therapy if she didn't have problems in facing psychic pain and putting her emotions into a symbolic form. Hence, however defended or hostile she is in relation to the therapy, I view the primary problem as being a problem of how I, the therapist, remain open to my own emotional experience with her and work on my countertransference. This would be as true for cognitive-behavioural ther-apy as for psychoanalytic psychotherapy.

Having a capacity to dip into the riches of my own emotional experience is essential. Some people are natural therapists, but many people, like me, require the rigour of personal psychotherapy or psychoanalysis to tap the reservoir of pent-up confused emotions. Left unrecognized, such emotions can distort communication between the young person and the therapist. For example, at times when I lacked sufficient self-esteem, I felt I deserved to be disliked by the young person and failed to understand the insecurely attached young person's fear of intimacy. Alternatively, needing reassurance that I was a 'successful and loved therapist', at times I was too weak, placatory and too charming to Marie. At these moments, I did not help Marie because I failed to acknowledge her split-off hostility in the transference which was being acted out in relation to family members. One of my biggest failings that I had to be alert for was an over-identification with Marie, which would lead me to be hostile rather than empathic towards her parents and their inadequacies in meeting her needs. For example, Marie would mention her mother shouting at her and I would get wrapped up in thinking about mother's inappropriate

shouting and fail to address how Marie was hurt, hostile towards and persecuted by me.

Working on the Marie's transference to me and my countertransference
responses is the essence of psychodynamic psychotherapy (Money-Kyrle, 1978).
At the beginning it was clear that she experienced me as an intrusive parent or
projected her unwanted resentful baby-self into me by enacting various situations
like keeping me guessing, waiting and ignored. In eclectic weekly psychotherapy
seminars with colleagues, who have cognitive-behavioural, cognitive-analytic,
Jungian, Freudian, Kleinian, as well as other individual and family therapy
orientations, we have found that it is essential to embody these concepts of
transference and countertransference in each of our different models of therapy.
What is different between me and my colleagues is the particular style with which
we use our understanding of these concepts. Whatever our theoretical approach,
we are particularly sensitive to the need for a reliable setting and a consideration
of the ruptures in the relationship with the child as well as separations and endings and how they affect the young people.

As the focus of this chapter is on individual psychodynamic psychotherapy, I
shall briefly refer to a range of crucial therapeutic issues regarding this kind of
work. In fact, throughout the chapter I shall be returning to Marie's story to illustrate many of the issues and concepts central to psychodynamic work with young
people who have eating disorders. Some of the crucial therapeutic issues include:

- The treatment frame.
- Duration of treatment.
- Suitability for psychotherapy.
- Assessment for psychotherapy.
- Aims of psychotherapy and the therapeutic method.
- Using dreams for initial assessment and ongoing assessment of ther-
  apeutic progress.

The treatment frame

The context of individual assessment and therapy for young people is crucial
Anyone treating a young person with an eating disorder must be closely allied
with a physician. A doctor should take medical responsibility for the ongoing
evaluation of the patient's physical condition. The psychotherapist needs to
have a clear set of guidelines for the minimum weight for the young person's
age and height and degree of physical ill-health that warrants hospitalization.

It is likely that during difficult moments in therapy, and during the therapist's holidays, the young person with an eating disorder may wish to diet and
discontinue therapy. This is part of her style of dealing with the psychological
pain of separation. She identifies with the abandoning therapist, stops feeding
herself and abandons the therapy. For this reason, it is irresponsible for a
therapist to embark on individual therapy without ascertaining that there is

an effective therapeutic link between the parents and a colleague who will be helping the parents to help the child eat and will assist the parents to help their child return to therapy at times when the young person finds it difficult to continue therapy.

In the initial, very ambivalent phases of therapy, it is not uncommon for a young person to stop therapy, engage in starving or bingeing, using laxatives, and exercising while at the same time fostering the parents' denial that the young person has a problem warranting therapy. Sometimes the young person may also hide weights or overload on water to conceal her true weight from the parents. Marie hid weights in a very secretive place, her vagina, and it went unrecognized for some weeks. It is, of course, absolutely essential to accompany individual therapy with ongoing work with the family or parents. Generally they want to find ways of being helpful parents to their starving child. That means they need help understanding their child's conflicts, containing her anxieties and firmly supporting their child to eat the required calories each day (Lock and Le Grange, 2015).

The most effective therapeutic frame I have encountered has involved:

1   At least two family assessments to ascertain strengths, weaknesses, and patterns of relating.
2   An individual assessment with the young person to ascertain the individual pathology underlying the eating disorder, bearing in mind that both anorexia nervosa and bulimia nervosa have typical behavioural patterns that conceal a wide range of emotional difficulties.
3   A medical practitioner to monitor weight changes regularly and to liaise with the parents and young person regarding the young person's physical health.
4   Parental or family work accompanying the individual therapy. This provides a better quality of support for the young person throughout life and enables the parents or family to find a safe context in which they can explore the problematic aspects of their relationships and develop their capacities.
5   Planning ahead by considering possible hospital provision in case the young person's health deteriorates. This is particularly important for those young people with severe difficulties, when they are faced with the initial holiday separation from the therapist.

Duration of treatment

Accepting the need for an adequate length of treatment is very important. Changing therapists is contra-indicated for an insecurely attached anorectic young person. It is also useful for the person doing the individual assessment to continue seeing the child, for even this transition from one therapist to another can be met with failure. Already filled with hurt, disappointment and rage about separations, prior to embarking on therapy, a young person doesn't find it easy to either change treatment services or trust another therapist in the same service after the previous one has left.

More than one eating disordered young person has expressed her fear, 'When I look all right on the outside, I am afraid no one will now notice how bad I feel inside. I want to be noticed, I want to be loved, I want to be very special to someone.' In saying this, Marie expressed her fear that, initially, she had to continually display her 'starvation' for fear that I, the multidisciplinary team and her parents would do as she did, that is, deny inner emotional states and focus only on weight loss and gain. I repeatedly needed to reassure Marie that she would be able to receive therapy until it was no longer needed. A minimum of two years is generally required to assist a young person to develop a stable psychic structure; however, this may not always be possible. Family therapy accompanied by a briefer period of Malan's (1997) focalized individual therapy or counselling can also be useful to enable a less ill anorectic young person to experience feelings in a more mature way and remain emotionally linked to others.

Suitability for psychotherapy

Because of the limited resources for individual treatment, and the efficacy of family therapy, individual therapy is often provided for young people who cannot develop their capacities for owning and containing their emotions through family therapy alone.

It is common for someone with an eating disorder to have disturbed psychic functioning involving the denial of painful emotions. This denial impedes taking care of the infantile parts of the self and thus prevents the development of emotional maturity. For this reason, individual therapy is potentially suitable for both verbal and nonverbal, motivated and unmotivated young people with an eating disorder. What is important is that the young person comes regularly to the sessions and the external network of professionals and parents support the treatment. The more crucial questions are:

- Is the therapist suitably qualified to work with this child's particular difficulties as well as having a compatible personality willing to tolerate the full brunt of the young person's projections of mental pain (Meltzer 1967)?
- Does the therapist have the willingness and capacity to work on the countertransference experiences to meet the needs of a young person who has not yet transformed bodily experiences into emotions suitable for language – for example, the silent, negative, or borderline psychotic young person?
- What help can be provided for a young person who 'closes her mind and mouth' to psychotherapy, as she transfers her starving and bingeing impulses for food to a rejection of the therapist or to a very demanding wish to be with the therapist all the time?

- What supervision/support is being provided for the therapist to work on treatment impasses both within herself/himself and the patient?
- If required, is the therapist skilled enough to avoid persecutory questioning and to use description, play, art and other creative activities to engage a young person in working on emotional issues when the young person is not yet ready to put words to her experience?
- Is inpatient or day-patient treatment initially necessary to support the young person in undertaking the burden of working through her difficulties?

Assessment for psychotherapy

Even if family therapy is the treatment of choice, each young person with severe problems also deserves the right to a private space apart from the family to think about her life and those issues that initially may be difficult to share with the family. It is not the young person's conflicts per se, but her capacity to think about them, to mentalize, which should be the primary focus of the assessment. The assessment process is fully described in Chapter 2.

Here are some of Marie's remarks illustrating her relationships to internal parental figures.

> My mother isn't able to understand me. There is no point in talking to her, she just gets upset.
> My father vents all his anger on me, not on anyone else.
> My sister is a 'greedy pig'. She gets everything she wants.
> If I had to depend on my parents, I'd commit suicide.

Marie was explicit in showing that at that moment in time she was dominated by internal parental figures who could not be depended upon, who did not understand. She projected her own feelings into her 'angry' father, 'greedy' sister, and 'non-understanding' fragile mother. The parental figures take little responsibility for potentially overwhelming feelings such as greed, jealousy, anger, and the incapacity to understand feelings in herself. The child-part of the personality feels so antagonistic to the parental figures that she would prefer to manage without them rather than face the frustrations of depending on them. Perhaps most striking was the inability of Marie to face the problems of relying on her parents.

When I attempted to look at Marie's capacity to look at her distress, as well as her capacity to struggle and be curious about her emotional life, I learned that Marie was reliant on her own omnipotent methods of taking care of herself. By this I mean she was reliant on controlling activities involving concrete activities such as dieting, counting calories, and exercising, rather than relying on either her parents or an inner capacity to have empathy and tolerance for her own emotional experiences. Denial rather than mentalization was her method of dealing with any issues that were too intense, too painful and/or too terrifying.

The psychotherapist needs to assess the severity of the self-protective structure represented by the child's omnipotent belief: 'I can take care of myself through physical and emotional dieting or through bingeing.' The stronger this defence, which represents a fragility in the underlying psychic structure, the more likely that, as therapy progresses, there will be crises during separations and holidays. I have earlier highlighted how vital it is to have a supportive therapeutic team of parents and professionals to contain the young person and support the therapy and the young person when the therapist takes holidays.

After four initial assessment meetings, if the therapist or young person really do not want to work with each other because of their personality traits, then neither should be required to be together. The meetings will be counter-productive for both parties. This incompatibility between therapist and child should be differentiated from a process which occurs during the course of treatment when the young person's hostility projected into food and her body and the hostility about separation, jealousy and other situations, will be transferred onto the therapist turning the therapist into 'the disliked one'. Parents and the clinical team need to be aware that this is part of the transference of hostility onto the therapist and it will create periods when the young person wants to stop or avoid therapy. In my mind, negative transference to the therapist during the course of therapy should be differentiated from a process in the initial phase of therapy when the two personalities of young person and therapist are not matched sufficiently well enough to commence work together in a collaborative way.

Aims of psychotherapy and therapeutic method

A psychotherapist's task is in many ways similar to that of parents. For this reason, psychotherapy is not a mode of treatment in which young people must have good verbal capacity or intelligence. Equivalents of the parent-child relationship include a focus on the young person's inner experiences including phantasies and dreams, the relationship with the therapist representing internalized parents and relationship with significant others. Also, the therapist, like the parents, needs to provide consistency of care, specific and defined boundaries to his/her body and the therapy room, as well as acceptance of the child even when she is destructive or rejecting. Also, a reliable and regular framework of meetings at the same time each week, with the same time allowance for each session, and sufficient preparation for therapy breaks, allows the child to develop trust in the therapist.

An enormous amount of goodwill, emotional availability and resilience is required for a therapist to be 'good enough' for the young person to develop through therapy. The therapist needs to be deeply attuned to the emotional experience of the young person, to give meaning to her communications. This is similar to a mother using her own emotional experience, coupled with her thinking, to make sense of the baby's expressions of physical and emotional states. Emotional attunement accompanying this mentalization process (Fonagy et al., 2004) is particularly important to remember for a young person with an eating disorder usually lacks integration of her physical and psychological experiences (Winnicott, 1958).

Because such lack of integration may be linked to a mismatch in communication in her primary experiences with her parents, a young person with an eating disorder needs the therapist to consider her very early infantile experiences expressed in the young person's demeanour, including sensations and movements of the body as well as hand gestures and facial communications. The therapist must do this before the young person can put her experiences into a symbolic form for communication. Only then can an integration of the physical and psychological self occur (Farrell, 1995).

Particularly at the beginning of therapy, the eating disordered young person often projects unbearable emotion and physical experiences onto the therapist before being able to feel, let alone verbalize, the experience. For example, hunger, nausea, tiredness, physical discomfort, anger, and sadness may often be first experienced by the therapist. The therapist then uses her own physical and emotional experiences felt in the presence of a child to understand these projections. If this acceptance of the child's projections does not occur, and the therapist just stays with an intellectual stance, the patient can get anxious (Dosamantes, 2004). The essential therapeutic task is to share the entire experience of the young person, empathizing with as much of the child's inner feelings as she will allow. Rather than intruding with questions or comments to the young person, it is often appropriate for the therapist to speak 'with the young person's voice' suggesting that the young person's nonverbal communication has been understood. For example:

> Marie was silent, face turned sideways with her hair hiding her eyes. She briefly glanced at me before retreating to look at the picture on my desk. I described the debate inside her: a debate about whether she talks with me or stays quietly alone. I also discussed how it seemed as if I were expecting something from her, and that she had told me she didn't want to talk with me. 'Yes,' Marie said dismissively. I replied that she spoke as though I really was a nuisance. I added, using a loud and angry intonation, as though I was speaking with Marie's voice, 'Things are all right. Let them be. Don't upset me by talking about something. It just causes problems.'
>
> In response Marie began talking about how the maths teacher always shouted at the people in the class. Only later was she able to admit being angry with me. I described how Marie wished that I would simply listen to what she was saying and think about it. Then I commented on how

she had experiences that she felt unable to put into words, and I felt she wished I could experience her depth of feeling without her having to put it all into words for me. Marie nodded affirmatively.

Healthy psychological development can be ensured only through the presence of an effective inner psychic structure, functioning as parents' understanding the emotions of a young person and inspiring hope for the future. Through the therapist's work of bearing feelings and giving them meaning, the young person can begin to experience being understood and accepted. This experience and further experiences of being helped in this way can then be internalized in the inner world of the young person to form a resilient mental structure for transforming unbearable sensations into feelings suitable for thoughts. The structure is designed to 'hold in mind' these intense and/or unbearable loving, hating, and conflictual feelings until thoughts about them can emerge. This process of holding feelings in mind and thinking about them is called *mentalization* (Fonagy et al., 2004). It involves identifying and naming what one is feeling, modulating it to give it more intensity or duration depending on the circumstances required, and then, through thinking about the emotion, choosing a suitable mode for expressing the feeling, either outwardly to others or inwardly to oneself.

Using dreams for initial and ongoing assessment

Regardless of their underlying difficulties, in the course of their therapy, eating disordered young people tend to progress through similar phases of emotional development. This developmental course is well illustrated by the young person's dream-life which functions as a kind of internal theatre with internal family figures entering into emotional relationships and conflicts with one another (Meltzer, 1984).

Stable developments, the growth of the personality's inner strengths including the capacity for mentalization are most reliably traced through assessing the dream structure and the young person's emotional relationship to her dream experiences (Magagna, 2005). At present, the study of psychic development as observed through the dream process is a poorly researched area, yet the dream and the young person's relation to it potentially presents one of the clearest pictures of the young person's developing emotional capacities.

The dream structure of the young person in therapy suggests a fluctuation in development of maturity in the dream which includes a sense of responsibility for the feelings expressed in the dreams and a capacity for mentalization. One can view the dreams as unconscious thinking, equivalent to the action and play of young children. As the young person discusses her dream, the therapist can focus on how the mind copes with emotional experiences, and how it deals with the distortions formed by the conscious self during the day (Meltzer, 1983). The focus of the therapist's interpretative work is to help the young person look once again at her relationship with the parental figures as re-enacted in the relationship with the therapist. There is a gradual demarcation between the infantile feelings of the young person and more mature parts of the young person's personality. Maturity is characterized by taking responsibility for thinking about emotional experiences and a growing acknowledgement, loving concern, and sense of responsibility for destructive feelings and actions.

The phases of the eating disordered young person's dream-life reflecting psychic development seems to follow this sequence.

- There is difficulty in remembering dreams and/or difficulty accepting they are meaningful. 'I don't dream' is frequently stated in the first meeting with an eating disordered young person. This is a reflection of a rigid barrier between rational thoughts and the spontaneous expression of feelings which don't feel loving, rational and in control. The inability to recall dreams should change during the course of a successful therapy of any theoretical orientation.
- Dreams are described in which the young person is overwhelmed with feelings that take over her sense of self. Examples might be:

    – The young person dreams that she is a Porsche. She has completely lost her own physical identity as she becomes an expensive racing car. Or
    – The young person awakens from dreaming that she is disintegrating while falling off a cliff.

- Dreams are described in which the young person uses the omnipotent self as a means of caring for her distressed self. The destructive feelings previously projected into the body have now emerged into the psychological structure in the form of greedy animals. For example:

    – When the therapist is ill, the young person dreams that she is in a hospital with the therapist's face appearing and then disappearing. The young person is then left in a room in which big, fat cats and rats, as well as black, furry monstrous creatures, are coming out from cages. She is terrified. She then pets a black creature and says: 'Isn't it nice!' She has turned to a part of herself that gives her a perverse protection, but this is a false sense of safety, used to deny difficulties with separation from the nurturing therapist.

- Dreams have more human figures in them and unwanted feelings of the young person are projected into these figures so that they, rather than the young person, become the owner of these feelings. Meanwhile, the self is experiencing a sense of hating, but disowning, and being frightened of these feelings in others. The young person, in describing the dream, has not yet begun to acknowledge these disowned parts of herself. For example:

– She dreams there is a teacher scolding all the other young people in the class for being noisy and wanting too much attention.

• Dreams are described in which the young person projects her vulnerable feelings into others and, identifying with a parental figure, she takes care of her feelings located in others. At this point, the internal parental figure has developed the capacity for understanding and concern, but the young person has not yet fully owned her dependent, vulnerable feelings located in 'the others needing care'. For example:

– She dreams that a baby is falling off a cliff, but she has adequate life-saving equipment and is able to rescue the baby. She had previously reported the dream of falling off the cliff.

• The dreams suggest a more open acknowledgement of feelings in the self, but they are still uncontained and often seem to be on the verge of being enacted in the young person's external life. For example, in this dream the acknowledgement of baby feelings leads her to want to be looked after by her parents; however, instead she identifies with her parents' intercourse by getting into her parents' bed with a boy. She is confused between wishes for to have the baby-self held, comforted and fed and the wish to have the sexual intimacy of the parents. However, she has been able to dream, rather than act out these confusions through sexual behaviour as she had in the past:

– She dreams of getting into her parents' bed with a boy and then having a huge feast prepared by her aunt.

• The dreams suggest that not only is the young person more openly able to acknowledge her own feelings and locate them in herself, but also she is able to accept responsibility for her destructive feelings and show inklings of maternal concern both for herself and for her siblings. The feelings seem more contained, as though there is the possibility of thinking before acting on the feeling. For example:

– She dreams she is shouting at her mother while her mother is talking to one of the younger children in the family. Then she decides she can join in the conversation too. She doesn't need to interrupt it by shouting. Later she is playing on the beach with her baby sister.

• In the dreams there is a fluctuation between dependence on parental functions in herself and the therapist (representing understanding parental figures), and the use of the omnipotent self. For example:

—   She dreams she is in a snowdrift. She is cold and being pushed down
    by the weight of the snow. She keeps going, but then she sees a light
    and she struggles to reach it. In this dream there is a hint that turn-
    ing towards insight, in herself and in her therapist, might help her
    with the depression she feels as she acknowledges her loneliness.

•   In the dreams there is more frequent evidence of a developing capacity to
    acknowledge feelings, think about them and take responsibility for what
    they imply. There is a sense that the internal capacity to parent oneself, in
    identification with good parental figures, is being established. For
    example:

    —   She cries in the dream, feeling sad when she quarrelled fiercely with
        her mother. In speaking to the therapist about the dream, she realizes
        that she has been feeling more kindly towards her mother and treating
        her with more consideration. As she talks about this dream she is able
        to show responsibility for the punitive way she handles arguments with
        her mother. She describes how she is trying to reach some resolution
        of the conflicts.

By the termination phase of therapy, the young person is able to move from
the egocentric position of thinking only of her needs, to a position of protective concern for her 'baby-self' as well as her internal and external siblings
and parental figures. In this stage of therapy there is a continual struggle
between loving feelings and angry, hostile, jealous feelings. However, the
loving feelings tend to dominate the young person's relationships with others
as well as her relationship with her 'baby-self'. She no longer regularly
neglects her body or her feelings but rather she attempts to take seriously her
emotional and physical needs. Having internalized a mentalizing therapist,
she is able to truly 'parent herself'.

The initial phase of therapy: the total transference

Although it is essential for the psychotherapist to continually evaluate not
only internal psychic development but also ongoing external relationships
with family, school and peers, the scope of this chapter is limited to describing
psychotherapeutic progress and impediments to growth present in either
therapist or young person suffering from eating disorders. These developments or impediments emerge and are understood during the course of therapy through transference and countertransference communications present in
verbal and nonverbal communications which include physical sensations, tone
of voice, gestures, dreams, drawings and play or enactments.

Although as a therapist I am filled with willingness to offer hope and
understanding to Marie, she arrives being reluctant to be present with me.
She has been cajoled by her parents into coming first to an outpatient

assessment and then to the inpatient eating disorder unit. She feels 'too fat'. Her parents haven't told her she is too fat, but she is aware that there are girls thinner than her in the gymnastics class. Marie outwardly appears angry because her parents have brought her to the clinic. However, I am aware that this anger conceals fear of intrusion by the entire inpatient and outpatient eating disorders team.

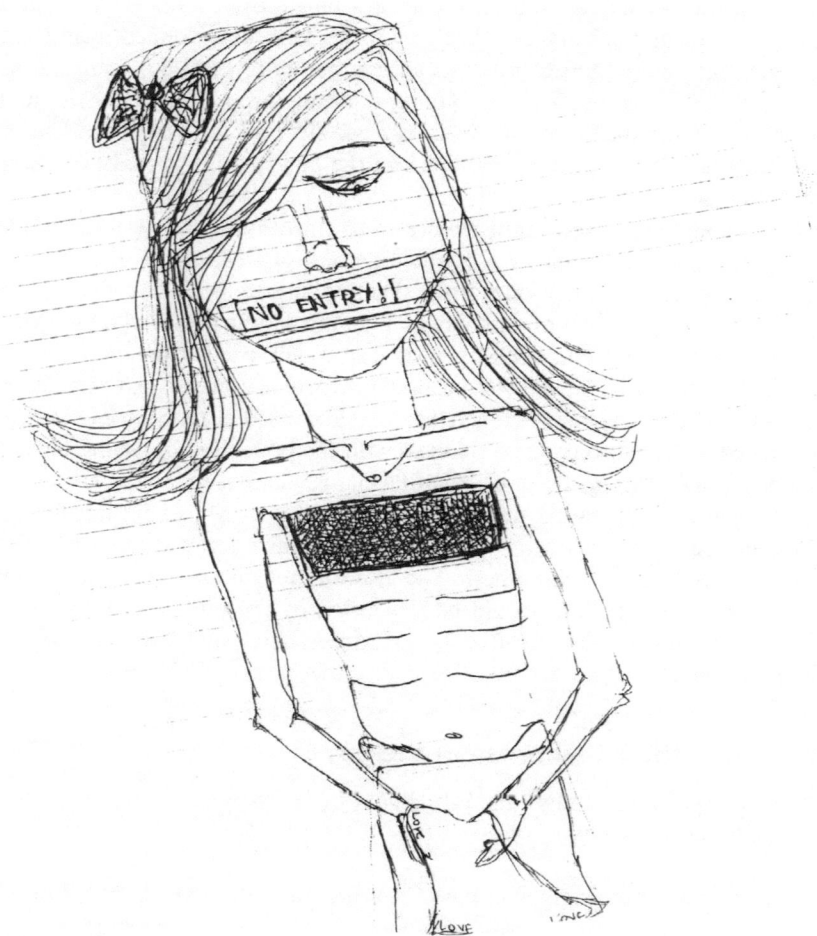

Figure 3.3 No-entry girl

Psychodynamic psychotherapy is characterized by a focus upon the 'total transference' of the young person to the entire institution, rather than solely to the individual therapist. By this I mean that the whole of the young person's current emotional response to the setting, staff, and institution procedures – such as physical examinations, weighing, and dietary advice – are gathered into the transference relationship to the therapist. In this context, 'gathering into the transference relationship' (discussed earlier) implies that the psychotherapist holds herself as representative of all clinical activity in relation to the young person and her family (Janssen, 1994). In gathering the transference with Marie it was also essential to look at her previous relationship with the paediatric unit where she had previously experienced an unsuccessful and fraught admission. While there she had been isolated from friends and the team attempted to offer social contact as rewards for eating, a task that she didn't accomplish and perhaps found impossible. This led to an increase of resentment towards both her parents and the hospital. 'The problem is that I am fat and my parents and the nurses want to make me fatter,' said Marie.

Understanding her total transference to the institution meant understanding that Marie felt threatened by the whole pattern of treatment – the intrusions through physical examination, family therapy, and re-feeding in the inpatient unit, as well as the threat of intimacy and understanding provided by individual psychotherapy (Magagna, 1998). Marie desperately needed me to understand that her 'delusion of fatness' was a bodily experience, which felt terrible. She had 'fat', which she knew spoiled her self and needed to be controlled and eliminated. Marie also equated thinness with the possibility of feeling beautiful and being liked by friends rather than feeling isolated at school.

Like many of the eating disordered boys and girls, Marie did not fear getting tall. In fact, she wanted to be taller. I felt Marie equated tallness with an inner bone structure holding flesh. She also did not mind having hard bulging muscles because her flesh would be structured by the muscle. It was the 'fat' without any inner structure that bothered her. And she feared we were all trying to make her 'fatter'.

Dreams in the initial phase of therapy

Marie brought several nightmares, typical of this first phase of therapy. These included the following:

> Marie awakens at night because of a nightmare consisting of a horde of people banging on a wall to come in. She sees a crack in the wall appearing as though they may be successful.

And

> In her nightmare, the shadow of a huge man is falling on the wall and she can hear footsteps as though he is about to enter her bedroom. Marie awakens and cannot get back to sleep.

These dreams suggest that Marie has a physical sensation of occupying a space that is being intruded upon by sinister, destructive forces or people. She depicts herself as being vulnerable and weak, while being devoid of any hostile emotions. There is a sense that she sees herself as good and the horde as a malevolent intrusion. I wonder if the feelings split off and projected into her body and the intruders are threatening to arrive into her conscious mind.

Countertransference issues: the total transference

Marie is fixedly holding onto: 'I am fat. The only problem is that the hospital wants to make me fatter and that makes me feel terrible.'

As a therapist, I am wanting to share my understanding of how I think about the problem regarding 'feeling fat' and all the complex experiences which that implies. I believe that her repressed hurt, rage and hate towards people closest to her, for disappointing her, for not being exactly as she wants them to be in relation to her, create a sense of being filled with internal parents who are damaged by her rage and anger. Her body, a woman's body, is identified with that of her mother's. Hence, she occupies a body that is filled with hostile feelings and thereby damaged. Her body is not able to hold intense split off feelings or sensations in a manageable form. Therefore her body is felt to be ugly, fat, and lacking a solid internal structure. I also imagine that the previous dream displays how Marie has projected her destructive feelings onto the sinister invaders. I also wonder if she has been sexually or physically abused, since about 25–40% of the eating disordered young people have also experienced physical violence or sexual abuse. This needs to be addressed as soon as, but not before, Marie begins to trust some member of the team.

Marie continually laments: 'The hospital wants to make me fatter.' My countertransference is that she needs help and I wish to offer her help in the form of joining her to develop insight into the symbolic meaning of her dilemmas. But this would simply lead Marie to feel I am making her 'fatter', with more unmanageable feelings.

I thought then of Moreno (1914/1977, quoted in Goldman and Morrison, 1984, p. ix–x) who, when he was responsible for looking after very distressed refugees in an Austrian camp, wrote:

A meeting of two:
eye to eye, face to face.
And when you are near
I will tear your eyes out
and place them instead of mine,
and you will tear my eyes out
and will place them instead of yours,
then I will look at you with your eyes
and you will look at me with mine.

I realized that the 'exchange of eyes' in which I would look at myself and the hospital through Marie's eyes would involve inhibiting my counter-transference wish to rescue or nurture Marie through providing insight beyond that which she had already shared with me. So, I simply said to her, 'You feel you need to be in control. This control of fatness makes you feel safe. You feel you need to be in control of the situation here.' 'Yes,' replied Marie. 'I write down every calorie that I eat.'

In this initial phase of therapy Marie could only bear to hear descriptions of the ways in which she tried to protect herself from feeling anxious. Originally, when I offered what I felt were more insightful interpretations and they were rejected, I felt they were simply incorrect. However, when I saw Marie's eyes turned away from me, I realized that in my therapeutic zeal I was providing too much understanding, which simply threatened the existence of her omnipotent self, which she still felt she needed to 'hold herself together'. She needed deny her 'crying self' for it was a threat to her safety, her emotional equilibrium. I am reminded of this through the picture Marie drew later (Figure 3.2). In it there is a big lock closing the door to her mother, as though her mother, represented by me her therapist, is a threatening intrusion.

The main problem in the countertransference at this stage is that, while wanting to feel helpful and potent as a therapist, I am being imprisoned, restricted, and rejected as a result of barricades erected by her omnipotent self. Her omnipotent self exerts control through thwarting Marie's experiencing of difficult feelings and pleasurable moments in the intimacy of our relationship. At times it was inevitable that I experienced anger and frustration as I was rejected and imprisoned by the slowness of pace required by Marie. At times, I realized that Marie was communicating her hostile feelings by re-enacting situations in a way that I might experience the feelings which felt so overwhelming, frightening in their cruel intensity, and disliked in her own personality. As she turned away from me, drawing but refusing to speak to me, I was to feel 'the rejected girl, who felt isolated in school and disliked by her classmates'.

If a therapist needs to be liked by the young person and cannot tolerate the experience of being a bad persecutory figure and feeling retaliatory hostility about being rejected, there is a tendency to 'split the transference'. This means that young person will experience the therapist as fragile or idealize the therapist while showing hostile feelings to the parents and inpatient staff. This can lead the young person to act out in ways which may include physical aggression to the body or towards inpatient milieu or parents. Gathering the positive transference and allowing the negative transference to remain split off can occur for a variety of reasons. These include the following.

- The therapist has too great a need to feel loved by the young person or vice versa.

- Either due to a transference of a weak, damaged parental figure onto the therapist or because the therapist is not sufficiently strong, the young person feels the need to protect the therapist from hostile, destructive feelings. The young person is afraid of the therapist and afraid of the therapist not liking her if she is verbally hostile to the therapist.
- The therapist has not sufficiently integrated her own latent hostility and thus is blinded to the hostile, destructive aspects of the young person in the session.

Assessment of the eating disordered young person for borderline psychotic features (Lubbe, 2000) is particularly important before treatment emerges, for this is particularly the kind of patient whose split transferences can lead to severe treatment difficulties with even the most experienced psychotherapist, regardless of her theoretical approach.

When I hear stories of the young person giving presents to the therapist early in the treatment, while giving hell to the inpatient staff or parents, I become alarmed that the patient is latching on to the therapist in a very primitive 'skin-to-skin' way. This means that separation from the therapist leaves the patient feeling torn away, thrown away by the therapist. Many eating disorders in young people can be rooted in early infantile hurt and accompanying rage about separations from the primary parental figure. A mother may be weaning the baby from the breast, having another baby, separating in order to have time for sleep, work, or another person, like the father. Rage about unmet needs, but also a possessive rage and panic about separation from mother or a nanny, are often some of the fundamental issues to be addressed in a comprehensive way in working with an eating disordered young person.

In therapy the separation issues can be acted out by the young person who feels she has a good experience in the session with an idealized therapist but then goes out of the sessions with an internal image of a therapist who cruelly abandons her. During the interim between sessions, all inpatient staff or parents are then seen as representatives of the cruel, abandoning therapist and are treated miserably by the young person. It is for this reason that any kind of regular therapy requires that the therapist fully prepare the young person for separations and gather in the transference the variety of feelings about ruptures in the relationship, ends of sessions, holidays, and the ending of the therapeutic work.

'Gathering the infantile transference' in this way is necessary throughout therapy with an eating disordered young person who may often have previously existed with an insecure attachment to her primary caregivers. This is important not only in relation to crucial issues of separation, but also in relation to all the other themes the child brings in her stories. The therapist's task is to ask how the theme of the young person's story may be relevant to the therapeutic relationship at that immediate moment in the session.

For example, when Marie described how her mother always made her wait for ten to 30 minutes to be collected after her gymnastic class, I became aware that I was being invited to identify with Marie and criticize her too busy and thoughtless mother. (How much easier it is to identify with a child's grievance towards her mother, rather than oneself!) However, gathering the transference meant that I noted I was two minutes late for that day's session and she had had to wait three days since the previous session. I said,

> I seem to be a therapist who does not think of your having to wait for three days. Then you feel disappointed and angrier when I arrive several minutes late, walk by you in the unit, not offer you a session, but talk to the nurses instead.

A transference interpretation, such as the previous one, is a primary method of psychodynamic work, but by no means the only one. I also wondered with Marie how she might talk more directly to me and also her mother. I tried to explore her anxieties about talking directly about a conflict she was experiencing. I noticed that repetitive discussions regarding food intake and weight control, needing to lose or gain weight, often occurred at the very moment Marie and I were talking about conflictual issues which really mattered to her. I silently noted that when you depend on another person and need them to be available, one of the worst things is that you cannot control them. That is the problem with depending on another person. On the other hand, food intake and weight gain can be controlled. Obsessional control of the body often occurred when Marie was most frustrated and hopeless about working out emotional conflicts with me. We looked repeatedly at how she turned to omnipotent control, talking about in relation to weight, shape issues and obsessional behaviours and thinking, at moments when she experienced intense hostile, painful or loving, dependent feelings in relation to me.

Boredom in my countertransference often occurred when yet again food related issues were being examined. I discovered that at times Marie mind was 99% occupied by the world of food and dieting with the recurring omnipotent phantasy of being in control of 'a body'. She drew a chart to show me this fact. This was how she emptied her mind of intense emotions and conflicts in relation to me, whom she could not completely control during the session. Gradually we jointly developed some way of describing how Marie safely went back to her attachment to 'food talk' as a method of moving away from something difficult. For example, on one occasion, when we tried to explore together why the 'food talk' had emerged again, Marie said, 'I tell you something insignificant and you make a mountain out of a mole-hill. You make my problems bigger than they were in the first place.'

Middle phase of therapy: integrating of split-off aspects of the personality

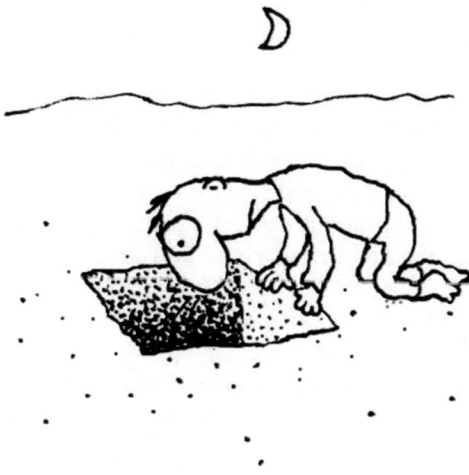

Figure 3.4 Let us listen to the heart (copyright Michael Leunig, 1990)

... Let us pause from thinking
and empty our mind. Let us stop
the noise. In the silence let us listen to our
heart. The heart which is buried alive. Let
us be still and wait and listen carefully. A
sound from the depth from below. A faint
cry. A weak tapping. Distant muffled
feelings from within. The cry for help.
We shall rescue the entombed heart. We
shall bring it to the surface, to the light
and the air. We shall nurse it and listen
respectfully to its story. The heart's story
of pain and suffocation, of darkness and
yearning. We shall help our feelings to live in
the sun. Together again we shall find relief
and joy.

(Leunig, 1990, p. 31–32)

The middle phase of therapy is characterized by Marie developing a deepening trust in my capacity to understand and accept her emotional experiences. My ability to do this is greatly influenced by my own willingness to remain emotionally alive to my own feelings and bear the psychic pain of accepting intuitive insights that Marie consciously and unconsciously highlights in my personality. For example, Marie said, 'I have defeated a famous consultant and I will defeat you.' Here she was aware of how her exploration of her own motivation was interfered with by my anxious wish to facilitate a successful therapy. I needed to try to deeply understand her. That is the primary aim of psychoanalytic psychotherapy.

As a psychoanalytic psychotherapist I was required to have an extensive personal therapy myself, to develop access, through dreaming and free associating, to both loving and destructive aspects of my personality and to develop the capacity to integrate as much as possible parts of myself that may previously have been projected. Yet, however much psychotherapy I, as therapist, have, there remain deeper conflicts and buried hurt (Figure 3.4), which can easily be projected into Marie or simply split off from the central core of my personality. The need to repair this buried part of the personality, and become what one truly can be, is part of the unconscious motivation for people choosing to work psychotherapeutically with young people having eating disorders which are most often accompanied by unintegrated, split off and projected intense feelings.

Marie's unconscious messages to me provided the most penetratingly honest and helpful supervision of my work to facilitate repair of internal damage both inside Marie and within me. The best psychotherapy is a 'duet for two', in which buried and undeveloped parts of both the young person's and the therapist's personalities are resurrected through the young person's neurotic and psychotic transferences to the therapist. Healing inside Marie became possible through the way in which I, with considerable patience, listened carefully to Marie's story of pain and yearning (Leunig, 1990), and developed understanding of her on the basis of understanding my countertransference. If the therapist does not develop in the course of being with a young person in therapy, it seems likely that the young person will reach some kind of impasse in the therapy. Then her spontaneity, creativity, capacity for intimacy, responsibility and thinking about her emotional life will not fully emerge.

It is a fallacy to assume that I can truly change another human being. My psychotherapeutic aim is to understand my countertransference responses which ultimately inform all that I am and do with Marie. I shall now delineate some recurring experiences in the transference and countertransference that have initially created an impasse but, through work in the countertransference, have facilitated development of Marie's internal psychic structure.

Six recurring problems

I have already mentioned that the underlying nature of various eating disorders varies and reveals a multiplicity of pathological states of mind. Despite this, there are some common challenges in the middle phase of therapy with a young person with an eating disorder. They are often present at different phases of the therapy, but it is in the middle phase of therapy, when the young person has become more fully known to the therapist, that the underlying pattern can be seen more clearly. Using clinical vignettes, I shall illustrate six challenges to therapeutic progress with Marie. The challenges include:

- Silence.
- Hostility, fear, and revenge.
- Rivalry.
- Obsessionality and intellectualization.
- Eating difficulties forming part of the transference.
- Placatory external progress masking inner difficulties.

Silence

I have only twice had the experience of treating a young person with an eating disorder without moments or hours of no words being spoken. There is always communication taking place between the young person and the therapist, but when the young person is not speaking, the therapist is particularly impelled to understand the prevailing mood derived from the posture and nonverbal gestures occurring in the therapist's presence and the therapist's conscious and unconscious responses to the young person (Magagna, 1996). If I, as a therapist in Marie's presence, can be still and in the silence listen to what is going on deeply within myself, then there is no need for me to penetratingly question her (Leunig, 1990).

During Marie's silences I have always felt that she required some silent space, lasting three to four minutes. I have never felt that I should be quiet for longer than that. She needed to feel that I was able to continue to reflect on the relationship between us and wasn't completely controlled by her silences. If Marie arrived and was silent, I often reviewed our previous meeting aloud, trying to focus on ways in which she may have felt understood or not understood by me. I also looked at her experience of the ending of the previous session as well as how it may have affected the space between the sessions. Most importantly, I have needed to decide carefully whether or not I spoke directly to Marie, or whether she required that I spoke in the third person. This involved my wondering aloud, not looking at her directly, creating a stage to the side of her, where I could explore the meaning of her emotions through a story or discussion with myself, with her choosing to listen or not listen. She needed to feel that therapy was not a recreation of being 'force-fed' by a controlling figure.

Because my countertransference responses to Marie's silence could seriously impede Marie's progress, it was essential to probe the depth of my own emotional response before venturing to speak. Outside the session, I would review the day in case my own issues or issues within the team were dominating and interfering with countertransference work of the therapy. If I did not monitor my own countertransference experience, I was unwittingly scripted into a counter-therapeutic role.

With Marie, it was useful during the silence to ask myself: 'Who is Marie being? What am I feeling? What am I supposed to be feeling in the role in which Marie has cast me? What is the meaning of Marie's drama into which I am being invited to participate?'

By using my countertransference responses, involving understanding Marie's feelings projected into me in the silence, I was able to give her the experience that unbearable feelings could be contained and thought about inside me. Gradually she was able to give her own experiences a symbolic form, sometimes first in a drawing and only later giving her emotions a name. Subsequently, perhaps much later in another session, she was able to consider them.

These were three main problems in my countertransference responses when Marie was silent:

- Firstly, I could feel too hurt and despairing about my ineffectiveness as a therapist, forgetting that I needed to use that sense of ineffectiveness to understand Marie's inner experiences of hurt, helplessness and hopelessness.
- Secondly, I could become overprotective, worrying that she wouldn't even come to the session if I didn't find some way of becoming just exactly the way she wanted me to be. This often stemmed from not sufficiently owning and elaborating upon my hostile feelings as part of what she was trying to communicate to me.
- Thirdly, I could get angry that she was not speaking and making my work easier for me, thus allowing me to feel I was in a helpful therapeutic situation with her. My wish to be 'a very good therapist' was dominating the therapeutic necessity of simply trying to help her think about and understand her emotions and integrate them within her personality.

These countertransference experiences created an impasse in Marie's therapy until I could transform them through understanding. To expand on and illustrate these points, here are some vignettes of repeated countertransference and transference problems in the verbal silences which occurred between Marie and me. They include:

- Overprotectiveness.
- Fear.
- Uselessness, rejection and despair.
- Need for primitive communication – heart-to-heart without words.
- Allowing separateness.

Overprotectiveness

Marie arrived and was silent. She had missed the previous session without calling to let me know she was not coming. I decided to ask her delicately why she had not come to the session. Marie responded, 'Sometimes I don't come because I am doing other things, while at other times I simply didn't feel like coming.' I didn't say anything more in response. It seemed to me she didn't want to discuss the matter further; her head was bent as though she was on the point of falling asleep and she did sleep momentarily. I remained quiet.

In this instance, I became too gentle and ineffective, over-anxious about hurting Marie's feelings in the course of therapy. Further examination of the countertransference made me realize that my gentleness was a counter-reaction to my anger that Marie never bothered to contact me and cancel the session or contact me after the session to explain why she hadn't come.

Fear

The child's need the omnipotent self's protective armour must be respected. For Marie, too much deep insight put too forcefully, or too 'emotionally intimate' interpretations, would often lead her to experience me as frightening. Overcome and threatened by powerful feelings, Marie would stop speaking as a way of protecting herself. She was holding herself together through silence. She didn't trust me. When I talked about her feeling that she had to have the protection of silence and respected her silence, Marie would sometimes spontaneously speak: 'You are always acting as though you know what I feel', or 'I feel miserable'. But when I attempted to speak with too much comprehension of underlying feelings, Marie would say, 'I don't want to know about my feelings! I am sick of them!'

Uselessness, rejection and despair

I had to admit that at times I was simply useless because I kept on saying the same old interpretation using the same imagery. It inspired neither Marie's curiosity nor interest and certainly did not foster progress. But Marie's silence was a real test of whether or not I would accept projections of her rejection, helplessness and inadequacy. I had to differentiate between Marie's powerful omnipotent self actively attempting to reduce me to impotence by silent, supercilious and cruel contempt and another process when, by rejecting me, she was actually trying to communicate an unbearable experience of being rejected herself. How could I differentiate these very different experiences? Bodily language gives a partial clue, but it is only through the emotional tone in the silence, heard in my countertransference, that I could really make a differentiation between these two different emotional states. A different relationship, coloured by more loving, trusting feelings, needs to exist before there will be a wish for understanding through projection of a painful sense of being rejected.

Once when Marie didn't speak for over five minutes (during which I spoke part of the time), Marie told me, 'I really thought you wouldn't have gone on a mid-term holiday just when I was worried about returning to school. That just shows that you really just care about yourself!' Here, the quality of Marie's silence made it obvious that she felt rejected by me.

Need for primitive communication – heart-to-heart without words

Marie was sitting in the waiting room with her mother. She had her back turned to her mother and tears on the brim of her eyes. When she came into the therapy room she was silent. She sat with her legs dangling over the chair, in a slightly sideways position in relation to me. It seemed that she was alive with painful emotions, suggesting that I should keep out. In this situation I waited in silence.

Marie needed a safe quiet space before tears fell from her eyes. It was important for me to be fully present experiencing the depth of her feeling. I did not assume that crying meant sadness, because it could hide a multiplicity of feelings. In fact, later when I described how tears could have so many meanings, Marie replied, 'I am sad because I am always angrily pushing my mother away even when I wanted her near me. I don't understand why that is.' I realized that this was also a common feature of our therapeutic relationship and after a pause I mentioned this.

Allowing separateness

Because of the seriousness of Marie's underlying emotional disturbance, sleeping difficulties, and serious eating disorder, her mother and father had become more and more overprotective. At the time of her referral, she was often either sleeping in her parents' bedroom or having one of the parents sleep near her bed in her room. Because of her own anxiety, mother 'watched her like a hawk', and when Marie was on the ward there were times that she required close supervision. Her enmeshed relationship with Marie had prompted mother to search her diary and drawers, discovering more about her sexual experiences with the older boys at school.

Therefore, it was important for Marie that therapy not be a re-creation of an intrusive relationship. She needed to know that I could be different from her mother and tolerate not knowing what she felt. Plying her with too many questions would also encourage her to be passive, waiting for me to take responsibility for the sessions. She might need to answer questions to please me, to allay my anxiety about her. I found that allowing some silence for a few minutes and exploring what she and I might be wondering about, without a question-mark ending my sentence, was often a more helpful way to be working in the session. This allowed me to think about Marie's experiences without pressuring her to feed me her thoughts at that very moment.

Hostility, fear and revenge

Minuchin's aim of helping staff and helping parents to work together (Minuchin, Rosman and Baker 1978) to provide firm boundaries and rules for the young person and help to the young person to eat is suitable for many young people with eating difficulties, but only if the parents experience compassion and sensitivity to the young person's terror. I have discussed how the more vulnerable, helpless, chronically starved, or emotionally disturbed young person may feel almost addicted to omnipotent self as a protection against an intense fear of losing a sense of herself.

Here is a dialogue Marie wrote regarding her relationship with her destructive anorectic self:

ANORECTIC VOICE: Food is weakness, the enemy. You don't need it do you? Anyway, food will make you FAT... even the smallest amounts. Food is not to be trusted. I am the only one who can be trusted. You can still live your life, go to school, go out with friends, as long as you obey me. You can, can and will be thin – skeletal thin, emaciated and go to school. Control is what you want.

MARIE: Yes, that is exactly what I want.

ANORECTIC VOICE: You are lucky that I came into your life and saved you – otherwise you'd be even fatter and bloated and GROTESQUE! Perfection does exist and you will strive to attain it no matter what. I am perfection. If you obey me then you too can achieve perfection. So are we friends then?

MARIE: Definitely. Forever.

Without the firm psychic boundary provided by psychic manoeuvres of controlling behaviours such as starving, dieting, exercising, vomiting and the use of laxatives, Marie felt as if she was exploding into 'fatness' or 'falling into bits'. Parents and staff need to bear that intense fear, and help the child feel safe when letting go of the anorectic self.

When behavioural procedures, including staff supervision of exercising and vomiting, were prescribed for Marie, she responded by cutting her stomach at night, hurling abuse, and hitting the staff. She also made an attempt to run away from the ward. The cutting of her own body could be viewed as her having turned away from us with hostility and then fearing that we could not be trusted to bear her rage without being revengeful towards her.

It was easy to notice Marie's violence, but much more complicated for staff to maintain a containing emotional stance experiencing not only her anger, but also her extreme terror. Marie was terrified because her entire protective armour was being broken into by the feeding process. As a result she felt her sense of self was being destroyed by the regime that said she must eat and not vomit. In other words, Marie's feeling was that her omnipotent self, struggling like a soldier in a combat field, was being destroyed by external authoritarian controls and that nothing would be left of her. Death, or superficially cutting herself, seemed to be the last weapons to which she could resort to win the battle of who was in control. Her attempts to die or harm herself not only symbolized her sense of her self being destroyed, but also portrayed her view that death was a wonderful relief from the terror of psychic fragmentation.

As I said, when Marie hit out, it was easier to be in touch with her aggression rather than her terror. There was an enormous need for the team and her parents to unite and bear despair, fear and anger and other uncomfortable countertransference feelings. When we were not successful in doing this, our rage with Marie for making us virtually impotent to help her was redirected to other staff members and the parents. Conflict within the supportive system around Marie then ensued.

In the therapy the focus was on Marie's collusion with her omnipotent self – the self that was fighting us to stay alive within her personality as her 'body-guard', but was actually cruelly taking away her life and destroying my and the staff's hope for her recovery. When I said this to Marie she responded, 'Yes, you are right!'

The omnipotent self was felt by Marie to be her only protection until she developed an inner psychic structure that was more helpful to her. At the same time she was terrified that it was forcing her to lose a helpful rapport with me and the adults who were trying to help her. Aggressive encounters provoking the danger of revengeful responses from me and the staff were an exciting camouflage for this primitive terror of the death of her physical and emotional connectedness to life, her primitive terror of psychological disintegration if she lost her omnipotent, anorectic self.

Rivalry

At times after Marie settled into the group-life of a ward and later when she developed a more dependent relationship upon me, both as an inpatient and while she was seen on an outpatient basis, rivalry with the other young people in psychotherapy with me propelled her towards being 'the illest child'. Unlike school, where the teacher notices achievement, Marie felt she could only be special to me by being a person who aroused acute anxiety in me and was therefore a problem. She felt that I was a therapist only because I was interested in problems, and particularly in anorexia since I worked on an eating disorder team; therefore, she consciously or unconsciously tried to cause me the most worry and most concern with the aim of being singled out by me as 'my special patient'. This pathological need to be 'the illest' through not eating and cutting, in competition with the other young people could have led to chronic difficulties, particularly when Marie was an inpatient. However, we worked on her maintaining an emotional connection with me between the sessions. This was done through analysing how her hostility about separation from me made me disappear as a supportive person. In this way, by keeping an internal supportive therapist, her need to be 'special' through being an acutely worrying problematic girl was reduced.

As the relationship with Marie developed, I became increasingly aware that, although I perceived her to be less depressed and to be experiencing more intimate relationships with friends and her family, she continually complained:

> Things are as bad as ever … I'm always a loner at school because no one likes me. I didn't do as well as the others on my school project … I am not ever able to talk to my mother as long as I would like, because she is always busy.

As I began to review the sessions in this context, I became aware that each time Marie discovered that a young person who was iller than her was admitted to the unit, the intensity of her complaints about 'things being as bad as ever' tended to increase. One day, she laughed with embarrassment as she told me that, while at the entrance of the hospital newspaper shop, she had 'accidentally' knocked over a younger, iller child whom she had pre- viously seen with me. Marie then told me, 'It's your job … from morning till night. You have patients, one after the other … until you are fed up … I wonder what I should tell you to get you involved … so as not to bore you …'

I realized then that Marie had to be 'a very ill young person' to keep me as worried about her as I had been when she was the newest and illest young person admitted to the inpatient ward. She was continually consciously or uncon- sciously in competition with 'the others'. No matter how much better and livelier she felt, I was to know she was 'miserable'. This was done to maintain the posi- tion of 'the most important young person', gaining most of my concern for her difficulties. She described it as her need to 'stick to me like ivy'.

Obsessionality and intellectualization

> …with a heart caked with cold past the brunt of feeling
> (Crowe Ransom, 1991, p. 37)

Control through dieting is used to stop eating impulsively, in an out-of-con- trol way. Phobias of certain foods, containing projected aggressive fantasies, may be present along with excessive dieting. Accompanying these sympto- matic behaviours are underlying phantasies which, when understood, lend meaning to problematic eating or vomiting patterns and the use of laxatives. Marie's mind functioned in a way similar to her eating style. When there was no adequate mentalization, which involves 'digesting' intense emotions through lending thought to them and integrating them within the psyche, Marie seemed to be on a 'mental diet' in which she avoided getting emotionally near certain crucial issues. An instance of this is the fact of Marie's sexual abuse. It was clear that unless Marie had brought up a particular dream, I might never have begun to talk about the sexual abuse by her older neighbour occurring over a two-year period. Until I noticed what was happening in her dream and discussed it with Marie, Marie had felt too guilty to bring up the issue of sexual abuse and subsequent sexual encounters with boys she met who were mainly using her for casual sex.

I also became aware that, in order 'to please me', Marie brought issues about her relationships with family members and dreams, in which she knew I was interested, because of the light they shed on her inner psychological situation. However, the reality was that, once her feelings were more obvious to her, she resorted to being emotionally distant from what she was describing. Alternatively, she blunted the emotional relevance of what she was saying, by running through a variety of topics without wanting to stop and allow either me or her to think about what she was saying.

Cold intellectual control was used to protect Marie from a torch of burning emotions which threatened her equanimity. So, for example, she reported with great calmness,

> Last night I was in an argument with my father. He lost his temper, pushed his fist right near my face and said he would bash my face into pieces, would throw me out of the house, if I didn't start being more obedient to my mother.

As she told the story in her cold, cut-off way, her feelings were projected into me and I was to imagine the scene and experience the feeling of terror and horror she regularly experienced at home. When things were really terrible, Marie's brick wall of detachment automatically arose.

'A heart caked with cold, past the brunt of feeling' (Crowe Ransom, 1991) is a necessary protection for a child to retain her sanity when she is overwhelmed by emotions which she cannot psychically contain. When I prematurely tried to look at Marie's emotional responses to her father, she simply spoke in a flat, detached way to me saying, 'I love him. This is the way he is and I have to accept that.' I learned from this that Marie's fear of some internal catastrophe led to a distancing of emotions by projection and 'intellectual control'. Until Marie's inner structure was ready to hold intense emotions, she could only gradually allow herself to be freed from the cover of cold intellectualization. Meanwhile, I was required to hold and explore the intensity of emotions within (Kennedy and Magagna, 1994).

Eating difficulties forming part of the transference

> If you spit in the air, it will fall on your face.
> (Midrash Rabbah, *Ecclesiastes 7:9*)

I have already outlined 'the treatment frame' for psychotherapy and high-lighted the role of parents who are usually asked to work together to help their child to eat. But it was easy for me to forget that, in the course of treatment, changes in Marie's eating difficulties were linked to the transfer-ence consisting of the developing relationship with me, for as her therapist I was now representative of Marie's internalized parents. My primary task as a therapist was to gather Marie's infantile feelings into the transference rela-tionship with me and free her from some of the unmanageable intensity of feeling that got projected onto her body and food and thereby interfered with her eating and psychological functioning. This was extremely important because Marie's depressed mother would simply have felt too attacked and shattered if she had been on the receiving end of all Marie's violent and ter-rified feelings that had become liberated during her therapy.

A consequence of 'gathering feelings into the transference' is that I had to accept the intensity of Marie's growing dependence on me as well as the brunt of her hostility. Marie trusted me sufficiently to tell me how hostility and fear dominated the process of getting better. She handed me a sheet with the tell-ing me what occurred simultaneously in her head when people said certain things to her:

Translations

1 'YOU LOOK WELL' means

- you've gained weight
- oh you're not thin anymore
- I don't feel threatened by you now
- I'm going to rub it in your face
- you are not ill anymore
- you're not anorectic

2 'YOU LOOK HEALTHY' means the same as above
3 'WELL DONE. YOU'RE DOING SO WELL' means

- you're getting fatter because you're declining anorexia
- you're not ill anymore
- you're gaining weight

   If anyone says these comments to you, then you are FAILING me. You, therefore, must, must try even harder to starve yourself, no doubt.

These were only some of the problems she was facing as she was beginning to look physically healthy. There was also the hostility, which had been split off and projected into food and into the internalized mother, resulting in Marie hating her body, which was identified with that of her mother's. When Marie was hostile to me, rather than accept her hostility, at times I retreated to feeling too guilty. I felt guilty when I let her down through misunderstanding, being too superficial or too deep, feeling hostile, and separating from her at the end of the session and during the breaks. Too much guilt led me into not being robust enough in looking at her contempt and hostility to me. A therapist who has not had sufficient psychotherapy himself/herself may become too defensive in relation to the young person. At times, denying my own aggression made it hard to accept the painful truth of just how hostile and contemptuous the anorectic young person can be. Yet it is so important to see and face this part of the young person to free her of the cruelty and perfectionism of the harsh superego within her. Similarly, without therapy oneself, it is often difficult for the therapist to realize just how vulnerable and dependent the young person can become once she appreciates her relationship to the therapist. However, until the therapist works through the young anorectic person's difficulties in forming a secure attachment and capacity for dependency on the therapist, the young person will overuse her protections of omnipotence, obsessionality and denial to cope with crises. It is for these reasons that I, as Marie's psychotherapist, required a supportive supervisory situation.

In the first phase of her therapy, although Marie began eating with slightly less difficulty, she had days when she approached me as though, the moment I opened my mouth, I was going to scold her or make her feel terrible. I had the sensation, at times, that my face was being transformed from Little Red Riding Hood's grandmother into the devouring wolf. There were days when the inpatient staff and later Marie's parents had to work strenuously to assist her to come to her therapy sessions. I had prepared them for the fact that 'terrible food' often gets transferred onto 'the terrible therapist' and that persecutory anxieties about food, now directed towards the therapist, could be understood in the therapy. But it was very uncomfortable to accept being transformed into a monster and very easy to believe that I was being viewed as bad by both staff and young person because I was an intrusive, inadequate, unloving therapist.

I realize now how important it is for me, and new therapists in particular, to accept that, although we do make therapeutic errors, for example, by not understanding or being too intrusive, part of the young person's negativity invariably stems from the situation itself. The point made earlier that young people with eating disorders tend not to choose therapy but are required to have it by their parents is significant here. In addition to this, some of Marie's negative feelings, once projected into the food, were transferred, particularly into my eyes, mouth and words and thus my eyes, mouth and words were experienced as intrusive. Words were felt to be equated with 'fattening food', and they made Marie feel worse at times, because the words helped feelings to arise inside Marie. My eyes were often felt to be sending rays of hate or depression into Marie to shatter her. My understanding was felt to be like 'dieting' which becomes addictive, controlling her mind and taking it over, so understanding also became intrusive and dangerous.

The thought that if you spit in the air it will fall on your face was helpful in describing Marie's transference relationship to me during the middle phase of therapy. Having made significant progress during the first term of therapy, I was shocked that, during my first three-week holiday, Marie lost several kilos. Later I realized that this can often occur in the middle phase of therapy when the young person appreciates the therapist and feels abandoned between sessions and during the therapist's holidays.

However, this occurred in the middle phase of therapy, for by this time Marie had developed a good therapeutic alliance with me. This meant that however much I discussed a change in the rhythm of sessions, Marie's response to separation from me was either consciously or unconsciously, generally one of feeling unsupported and unloved. Marie said, 'You just don't care about me. I always try to make my best efforts to please you, but then with you, like with everyone else, things always end like this … in being rejected.' Her 'spitting on me' for leaving her created an image of my being a bad, uncaring therapist. This feeling of my being a bad, hostile, witch therapist was 'the spit falling on her face' being relocated in the food, which then became more noxious to her during the holiday. Hence Marie lost weight.

But it was not only a therapeutic holiday that could create a significant fluctuation in Marie's acceptance of food. When her perfectionistic self demanded a perfect therapist and I didn't say something with quite the right level of emotional understanding or warmth, Marie became very cross. She would then say, 'Right, I'm not going to eat now.' She would then leave the session, keeping her mouth closed to food for hours and sometimes longer. Just as mother's food is equated with mother, so too does emotional food eaten during the course of therapy become associated with the therapist representing the child's relationship to her internalized mother. I gradually became confident that if Marie felt adequately supported by me internally, she would attempt to eat food no matter how difficult her experiences were. In doing this, I felt she would be identifying with 'a good mother' who felt her child needed to eat, no matter how unhappy or lacking in hunger the child was. Certainly Marie's experience was that, when she was filled up with anger or jealousy or unhappiness, she both felt 'full up' and also felt that the food was 'horrible, tasting like cardboard'. On these occasions her body also felt 'fat and disgusting'.

Gradually Marie and I developed 'a common metaphorical language' in which it was understood that her relationship with food was linked to her relationship with me, her therapist, representative of the 'parents-in-her-mind', the internalized parents. As we did this, I gradually stopped silently criticizing the parents for not adequately helping her to eat when there were 'blips' and instead began understanding the meaning of her not eating in relation to her transference to me. I now realize that Marie starved for many reasons including when she was angry with me. She starved to be in control of uncontrollable feelings experienced when outside the session, starved in identification with me starving her of therapy, starved instead of mourning the loss of different earlier developmental stages of our therapeutic relationship, starved because she felt fat when in trouble. That was her routine way of facing a problem when I or a parent wasn't around to help her with her emotional conflicts.

Placatory external progress masking inner difficulties

It is only with the heart that one can see rightly.

What is essential is invisible to the eye.
(St. Exupery, 1995, p. 68)

I have seen many a young person who has eaten to get out of hospital as quickly as possible and free herself from the nurses' eyes. The young person's aim in getting out of hospital was to lose weight again. The book *Anorexics on Anorexia* (Shelley, 1997) gives many accounts of feeding programmes without psychotherapy, which leave the young people feeling like this:

What really surprised and shocked me was the fact that the focus was on feeding me up to produce a change in my body, but never once did they take my mind into consideration. The way I was feeling did not seem important to them. I received very little in the way of counseling.
(Shelley, 1997, p. 3)

Although this may be partly a projection of the young person's state of mind onto hospital staff, a treatment programme that does not have stated therapeutic aims beyond that of weight gain promotes a distorted picture of psychological development both to the young people and to their parents. Likewise, young people can quickly work out what they feel is 'the right attitude' to get discharged from hospital. For those of us, parents or clinicians, who are prone to rely on the young person's comment: 'My weight is right now, everything is fine, now I should stop therapy', it is essential to remember that this is but the surface. Before making a decision to end Marie's therapy, I needed to understand her inner reality through listening 'with my heart' to her mood in describing her feelings. It was through the countertransference, accompanied by looking at her dreaming process, that I was able to ascertain Marie's capacity for mentalization, which would enable her to struggle with and ultimately integrate the destructive aspects of her personality. This process needed to be motivated by her love for others and for herself and also her capacity to bear rather than deny frustrations in the achievement of her personal goals.

When beginning work with Marie, I found myself unwittingly involved in the content of what she was saying about not wanting to eat, feeling everyone was controlling her, making her eat high-calorie food, and so on. At that time it felt essential for me to have the support of a supervision group. The emotional support of this group facilitated listening with 'a third ear' (Reich, 1948) to the emotional tone – a kind of accompanying music – in Marie's communication. This kind of listening then allowed me to begin to describe:

- How she was speaking.
- How I felt before, during, and after she was speaking.
- What my feelings revealed about her current inner state, often projected into me.

Recognizing a placatory tone and discussing it openly can often bring great relief to children in therapy. One creative way of exploring a counter-transference sense of 'placatory pretence' on the part of the young person has been shared with me by a supervisee (Neil, personal communication):

> I try to simply discuss the feeling of pretence directly with the young person. On one occasion then I tried to explore this, the young person said that the feeling was almost always there and that it spoiled every-thing for her. I suggested to her that the feeling of pretence might be linked to the angry feelings she tried to keep at bay. Using the image of a theatre set, I suggested to her, 'Every time "Anger" sees "enter stage right" in the script, the director (her) pushes "Anger" stage left and buries it in a box behind the set. Other feelings come and go, but with-out "Anger" the play is lacking. "Upset" and "Tearful" try hard to understudy but they are just not good enough. Not only that but "Pre-tence" (who is really "Anger" in disguise) insists on rubbishing every-thing else that goes on so the director, no matter how hard she tries, is left feeling awful inside.' The young person laughed at this, but I felt that she understood what I was getting at. She joked at the end of the session that she would think of ways of letting 'Anger' have a few lines now and then.

It is necessary for me to continually notice Marie's immediate response to my comment or interpretation, as did the therapist in the example. I say this because Marie's responses provided a means of ongoing supervision of my work with her. I could use her response to ponder over such questions as: Has my interpretation enabled her to feel:

- Accepted rather than criticized?
- Understood rather than penetrated with insight?
- Interested in further exploration of her emotional life rather than in control, which prompts retreat to superficial intellectual levels or attack on my interpretations?

Working well together as a clinic team creates an emotional climate which fosters a shift from intellectual exercises with Marie to a mutual exploration and mentalization regarding crucial issues. When the team was experiencing too much conflict, I found that either I or other team members working with her family reached an impasse. Our imperfect attempts to understand Marie and her family and our sense of impotence were not acknowledged as we simultaneously replaced these difficult experiences with criticizing Marie and her parents for various reasons, including suggesting they were 'not working' or 'not co-operating'. At these moments I realized that, just as parents sometimes direct unexpressed frustration onto the young person, so too does the clinic team direct their sense of impotence to the family members. Therapeutic impasses were quite likely to occur just at this time. When I or the family therapist decided to discuss a session with Marie or her family in our small supervision group, we were frequently surprised by how just the thought of working together with colleagues in this helpful and supportive way promoted a shift in our relationship with Marie and her family so that, not surprisingly, the next therapy session was 'not as stuck' as the previous one.

Expected changes: perfectionism, self-esteem, body image and body shape

An infant may use the body as a safe receptacle of hostility regarding the absence of a mindful, secure attachment figure (Spitz, 1965). For example, the infant may bang her head or hand against the wall or pick at her body. On the other hand, showing aggression to the caregiver depends on there being a reliably present caregiver who is trusted to receive the aggression rather than to strike back, a caregiver who, rather than being fragile, is sufficiently strong to endure the aggression without breaking down into tears, persecution and revenge (Stern, 1985). The continued use of the body to split off aggressive feelings to the primary caregiver, generally the mother, is perpetuated throughout life. Here are some statements showing how Marie used her body as an object of hate:

> I hate myself. I hate me. I hate fat.
> I hate the hospital. I hate the scales. I hate my body.
> I hate my body. I hate being judged by the number on the scales. I hate myself. I hate myself. I hate.
> FAT = ME WHY ME? WHY ME?
> WHY ME? WHY ME? WHY ME?
> Fat idiot. It's all my fault. I deserve everything I get.
> Messy, fat me!
> Fat and ashamed.

Not only is aggression split off into the body, but there is a sense that the psychological self can continue to exist regardless of whether the body is dead or alive. Young people with anorexia nervosa, such as Marie, have split off their aggression and projected it into their bodies. (Of course, a sense of a 'bad, disgusting body' can also be linked with physical and sexual abuse.) As their body approaches puberty, the various parts of the body still hold the projected aggressive feelings towards the mother and father. In such instances, identification with the mother and mother and father as a parental couple involves identifying with damaged parental figures, the 'ugly, fat and possibly disgusting' parental figures filled with projections of aggressive feelings.

But aggression from Marie projected into food and her body and her mother was not the whole story. As I mentioned earlier, Marie had also been repeatedly sexually abused for several months' duration when she entered puberty and she had kept it secret from everyone for several years. Having always had insecure attachments, she felt there was nobody she trusted with the information until she became an inpatient. Marie had used emaciation as her contraception method and finally, when she became skeletal, the abuser stopped abusing her. She hated breasts and a sexual body because she felt it just made her susceptible to getting abused. The abuse had heightened the sense she already had of a 'dislikeable, disliked, not good body'. Sexual or physical abuse or bodily trauma through injury, illness or hospitalization can also heighten this sense of a 'dislikeable body'.

In the first phase of therapy, Marie experienced her destructive impulses held in check by both projection of feelings into food and her body and denial of her destructiveness, due to the presence of a very harsh, punitive superego demanding perfection.

As well as straining herself excessively to achieve 'A stars, abstinence and anorexia', Marie also had to be a perfect good girl who loved people. The cruel perfectionist superego did not allow her to be conscious of any negative thoughts or feelings such as hurt, rage, anger, jealousy and possessiveness. Her omnipotent self didn't allow intense sadness from infancy, loneliness and unconscious longing for love to be known to her. As a result, Marie's façade seemed placid and cooperative in a placatory way as long as food wasn't the focus. Because she was so persecuted by a punitive perfectionist superego, she simply could not hold in her mind a negative opinion or hostile feeling towards someone important to her. Instead she would say, 'I am sorry.' But no one could understand what she was sorry about because they had not seen the hostile thought, buried in her unconscious.

As the therapy progressed, I became suitably safe for Marie to relinquish hiding behind the omnipotent self in order to turn to and begin to trust me. Then there was a flood of needy and destructive feelings which first emerged in dreams of wild animals, dogs and cats coming out of cages. It was as though the icy defence surrounding her personality was melting. As I began to differentiate and think about the wild animals, representing Marie's returning destructive feelings, Marie gradually was able to integrate her hostile feelings and consciously direct them to me. As she became more trusting and dependent on me, there emerged jealousy of the iller patients, the healthier patients, the patient just seen by me as well as possessiveness towards me for ending the session to go home to be with my partner, family, friends and work. What was essential was that I received Marie's aggression, give it a name and thought with her about its motive and effect on our relationship. Psychoanalytic psychotherapy aims to gather the young person's intense infantile feelings, including aggression and love into the transference relationship. Gradually the young person's destructive feelings are expressed and integrated with love for the understanding and reliability of the therapist. Subsequently the internal images of the parents change to those of supportive parents. This can be seen near the end of therapy in Marie's dream of a loving parent comforting a crying child.

This siphoning off of aggression from the external parents and internal parents and directing it towards the therapist, who can receive the aggression and understand its meaning, not only leads to different, more loved and therefore more benign, internal parental images, but it also then leads to identification with more benign parental figures. As a result, gradually the young person's body self image can become more attractive and this led Marie to begin to dress in a more age appropriate attractive way. This was suggested, near the end of therapy, when Marie drew the attractive young woman shown at the end of this chapter. Self-esteem is also based on identification with parents. Marie's self-esteem and body image could improve with the integration of aggression and love.

Likewise, as more benign, supportive internalized parents developed within Marie, there was a gradual lessening of her obsessionality which had been used in lieu of good mentalizing internal parents to support her and modulate her intense loving and hating feelings. Also, the cruelty of her perfectionist self was gradually being replaced by an inner capacity for mentalizing. These internal structural changes in Marie's psyche created a lot of anxiety. For a short while, in the absence of anorectic symptomatology, Marie became more obsessional as she felt that she was really losing a tight grip on her omnipotent, anorectic self, her protector against mental pain. However, as identification with benign internal parents was more consolidated, and as time progressed, Marie began to feel more positive about having a female body. She developed the capacity to experience pleasure in having a nice, sexual body, rather than a disgusting body. This was reflected in a capacity to use her body in more spontaneous, relaxed ways through dancing and volleyball. She also became interested in a boy who was loving and sensitive towards her.

The ending phase of therapy

> Won't there be at last
> For the things that are,
> Not death, but rather

Another kind of ending,
Or a great justice-something
A bit like pardon?
                    (Pessoa, 1917)

As for all eating disordered young people, separations and endings were an issue throughout Marie's therapy. Together we had to look at her responses to the limits of my understanding, which prompted her sense that I didn't care enough about her to understand and was dropping her emotionally. We also had to examine her response to the ending of each session, particularly when, just at the end of a session, she remembered a dream or felt she was just opening up in an important discussion with me. At these times I was to also hold her frustration of the ending of a session. Alongside these ending issues there were also the session endings which were followed by a holiday. Holidays had inevitably been accompanied by Marie feeling the rage about separation and anxiety about whether or not I would keep her in mind during the holiday. When she felt dropped by me she often identified with me as an abandoning therapist who left her starved of care and understanding. Initially this prompted her to starve her body some of the time so that she lost weight.

Marie experienced difficulties in elaborating on her rage with me and developing a capacity to care about me enough to allow me the freedom to be with her and have my freedom to have a necessary break from her. In view of these difficulties with endings, it seemed inevitable that when I agreed with Marie that in six months, on a definite date, her therapy could end, although her mature self felt ready to end therapy, termination of therapy reawakened old separation issues she had during different phases of her life in relation to her parents and me. In her infantile self, in contrast to her more mature self, therapy evoked rage about separation and a fear of being lost without me. For example, Marie brought a dream:

I was climbing a hill. For some strange reason it was all red. It looked a bit unnatural. There had been an explosion. I then found myself wandering around at the bottom of the hill lost.

In the ending phase of therapy, I encouraged Marie to associate to her dream and then try to make her own interpretations as she would need to do when therapy ended. She said that she felt the red might be linked to anger, the furious rage that she experienced being left alone. She worried that if she became too angry with my ending the therapy, she might end up feeling lost, with no good connection to me inside herself after therapy had ended. She realized that she had become dependent on the understanding provided in the twice-weekly therapy sessions. At the end of therapy there was the problem of her rage with me for not being 'an everlasting therapist', like her 'everlasting food machine' (Figure 3.5), which she drew earlier in the therapy.

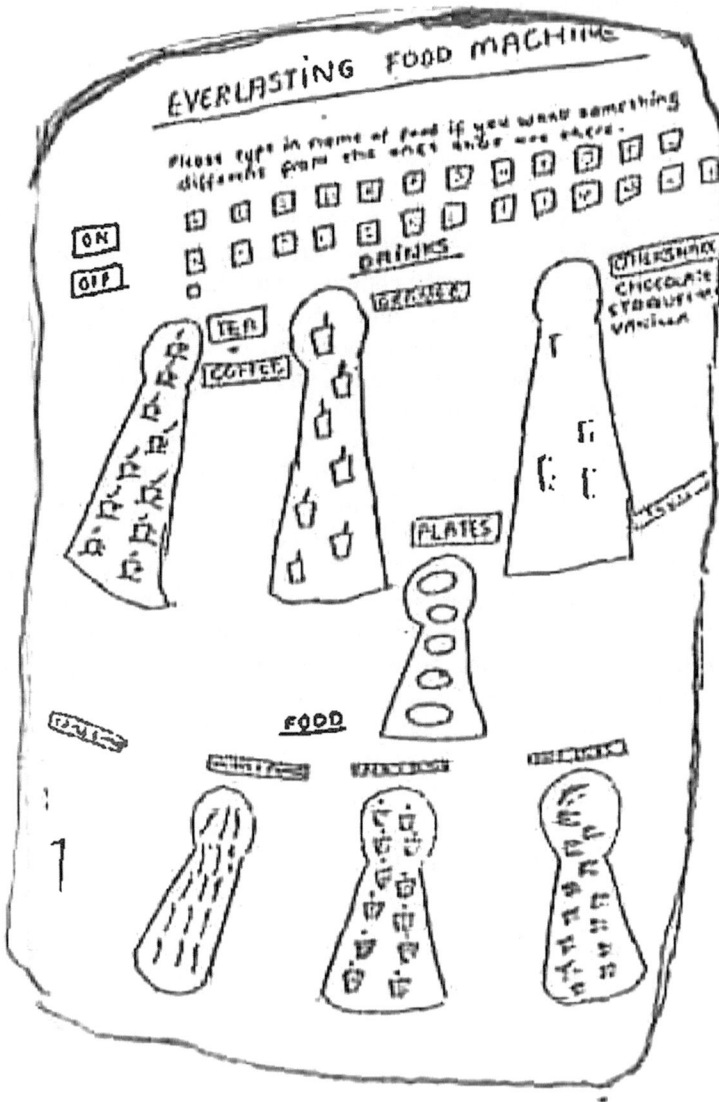

Figure 3.5 Everlasting food machine

I felt Marie understood her experience and described how it was being able to understand her internal experience and think about it which was the capacity which she took with her to continue developing outside the therapy. Nevertheless, she said, 'Strangely, I am tempted to diet again.' In fact, she lost a kilo right after this session. She also said, 'I sense that I am really tempted to get back into my rather non-stop jogging, but I know that is just running away from feelings and feelings can't be avoided forever.' I talked about the reoccurrence of some of her old issues, saying,

> This is a challenge for you. Can you think about the rage, rather than place it inside your body towards the me inside you? I understand now how when you feel overwhelming rage with me, your breasts and tummy feel 'fat'. You experience an ugly 'fat and fullness' of rage. Your body, identified with my body, feels exploded and in an ugly, damaged state. I can see why you then feel tempted to diet and jog.

Crucial in this ending phase, for which we had allowed six months, was a re-elaboration of certain themes which included working on:

- Marie's rage that I was not under her control like an everlasting food machine and her realizing that food and sex would not compensate for an understanding therapist. I was aware that when Marie was able to directly express her rage and disappointment towards me, a change occurred in her cruel, perfectionist superego that was so harsh and demanding of her. Integrating some of her destructive rage with me with her love for me drained the 'perfectionist voice' of some of its cruelty. Being so perfect at everything was then not so important to Marie as trying to use her capacities as well as she could.
- Marie's love and appreciation for the work of mentalization which we had done together to help her develop an inner capacity for using her intuition and capacity for mentalization.
- Marie's sadness about losing the therapy. This was initially expressed in this dream: 'I am looking after a little eight-year-old girl who is crying.'

But Marie's future stability was dependent on how she internalized the therapeutic relationship, a relationship never totally under her control. Stability and continued progress into her adult life would depend on how Marie continued the process of discovering and thinking about aspects of herself that emerged in her relationships by day and were portrayed in her relationships with internal figures in her dreams at night. To consolidate some of the work which we had done together in therapy and foster an internalization of the mentalization process, I suggested that Marie continue an ongoing structured inner dialogue through self-analysis done through a journal written at intervals similar to her therapy sessions. In this diary which she shared with me on occasion there was reference to a future which involved university, friends, a husband, children and a professional career. Her improving self-esteem was still filled with preoccupations concerning: 'Am I good enough? Have I upset anyone?' There was still much work to be done in her self-analysis. There was still the question of how capable she was of genuinely loving. Her sense of being deprived and her hostility continually threatened her developing capacity to love another person. However, this process of remembering her dreams, keeping a journal and developing a sense of mindful reflection assisted her in being truthful with herself and assisted Marie's mourning for the therapy space, which ultimately she had been able to use.

Two follow-up sessions, at a time of her choice in the following several years, were part of the termination plan. Marie returned for a follow-up appointment some years later. She had maintained a healthy weight and was eating normally. Finding pleasure in her studies as well as her friendships, she was able to communicate much more openly both with her parents and her boyfriend. However, Marie said she was always aware of the pressure on women 'to be thin and beautiful'. I felt that Marie's therapy had been helpful to her.

Successful therapy with a person suffering from anorexia nervosa involves providing a secure setting in which the young person can explore the full range of her feelings in *the here and now* in relation to the therapist. In doing so the task is to jointly develop an understanding of the young person which evokes gratitude and an attachment to the therapist. These reawakened feelings of love and gratitude, which had been split off and lodged in the anorectic young person's 'body feeling fat' became more integrated with the destructive, hate, rage, anger, and jealousy towards the therapist representing the internalized parents. A predominance of letting go of the destructive omnipotent self and relying on an internalization of the therapist's capacity to mentalize (Fonagy et al., 2004) should occur before the young person ends therapy.

Ultimately the young person finds a way of accepting that her parents and therapist are who are who they are, with their good qualities and deficiencies including lack of goodwill towards her. When she is able to forgive the parents and therapist for not being perfect, but rather being humans with frailties and problems of their own, she is allowed to hold better internal parents with whom she can identify both emotionally and physically. Her body becomes a vessel for loving feelings integrated with hating feelings. As such, whatever its physical appearance, her body-self can be experienced as having a certain beauty. Figure 3.6 shows how, once the split off aggression is removed from the body, concretely representing the mother, the body can be allowed to have its sexuality, its beauty and be treated with loving care.

The young person can begin to take more autonomous responsibility for looking after herself, including achieving proper weight necessary for menstruation, and developing friendships outside the family while remaining intimately connected to her parents or important caregivers upon whom she depends. However, at times therapy may also involve separating, at least temporarily, from parents whose problems grossly interfere with the child's psychological development.

Conclusion

Individual psychodynamic psychotherapy is costly in the short term because, with a child with a severe eating disorder, it is not something that can be

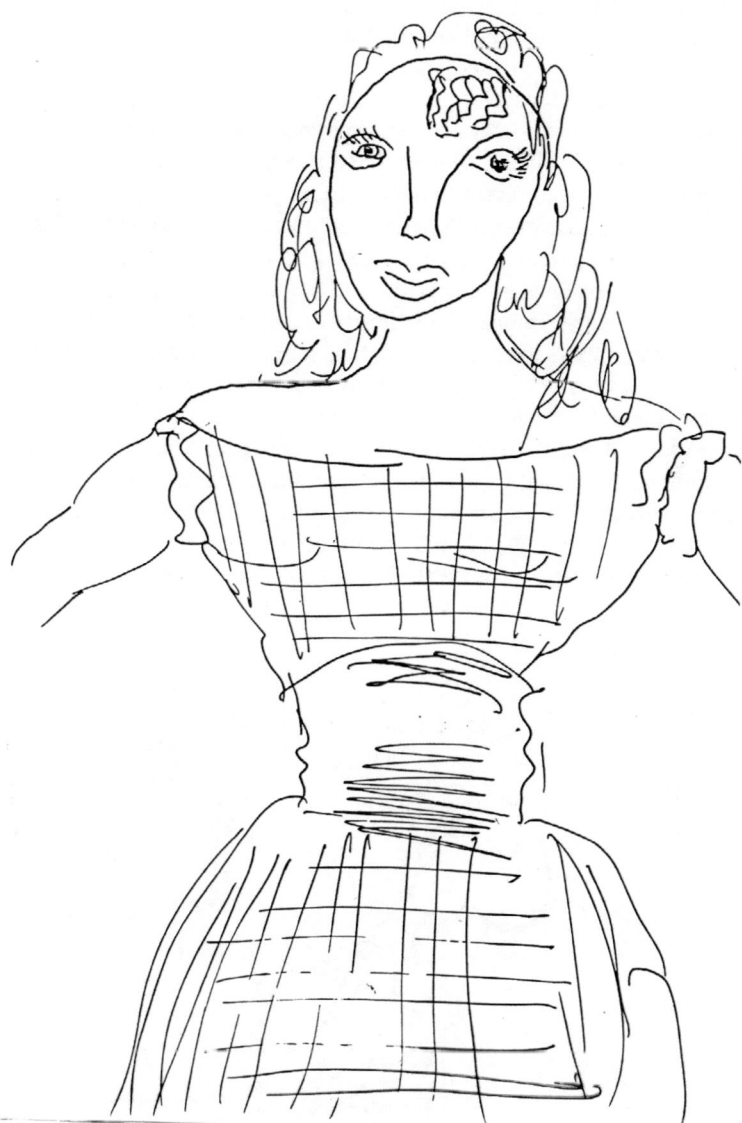

Figure 3.6 Drawing of an attractive young woman

successfully completed in six months. It takes time for the young person to begin to think about her life and develop a meaningful understanding of her symptoms. It takes time for the young person to move from a position of the self-protective, but ultimately destructive, omnipotence of anorexia nervosa which evades psychic pain to move to using a capacity for mentalization which involves bearing psychological pain. However, if the therapist and child are able to sustain a good therapeutic alliance to work through some of the child's central conflicts, psychotherapy provides a substantial base of security for the young person and for the psychological well-being of the next generation of children. When a young person leaves therapy, I regularly ask myself: 'What kind of a parent will this young person be?'

My therapeutic endeavours with Marie were to enable her to own within herself, rather than project, parts of her personality and unresolved emotional conflicts onto her body-self or onto others. Without therapeutic help it would certainly be very difficult for Marie to bear the intensity of her own possessiveness, hostility, and intense love in years to come. Left untreated, a mother who has suffered from anorexia nervosa of necessity can resort predominantly to denial of conflict and omnipotent methods rather than containment of anxiety when raising her own children. Also, left untreated for her anorexia nervosa, a mother may find her children difficult to parent for her own unmentalized emotions can easily be projected into them. And so we see another generation of difficult lives (Stein, 1994).

Hope for the future generation relies on psychotherapy for eating disordered young people to provide this:

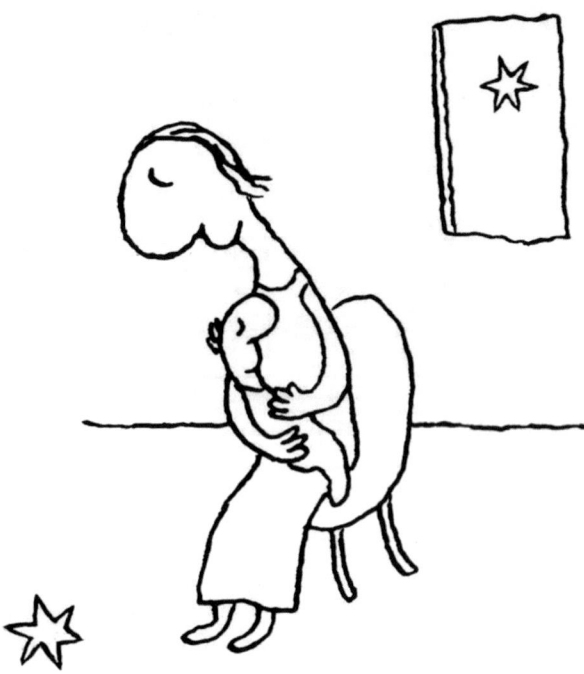

Figure 3.7 The mother holding a child

As she carried
her child may she carry her soul. As her
child was born, may she give birth and life
and form to her own, higher truth. As she
nourished and protected her child, may she
nourish and protect her inner life and her
independence. For her soul shall be her
most painful birth, her most difficult child
and the dearest sister to her other children.
(Leunig, 1990)

A good outcome for Marie, or any other young person having psychodynamic psychotherapy, would be a realized capacity to become an adult who maintains an intimate and mindful connection with her own emotional life and that of her children. This process of developing intimate mindful connections involves acknowledging both one's love and one's destructive feelings as well as developing a capacity not only for oneself, but also for others. To do this, the young person, through the supportive understanding of a therapist, must be able to move from a position of revenge towards the parents to a position of forgiving the parents for not being 'perfect' but rather being human with frailties and problems.

Chapter 4

Family therapy with a boy with eating disorders

Introduction

'I want to grow tall, but I also want to lose weight.' These words typify the problems encountered by an anorectic boy, Riccardo, and his Italian family living in London. In this chapter, I shall describe my work as a child and family therapist assessing an anorectic boy and then progressing into the family work of trying to understand and facilitate the development of the family members' Inner Child and their more mature capacities for mentalization.

The focus of this paper is differentiating two types of tallness:

- Tallness and growth based on omnipotent functioning in identification with 'super-parents' designed to evade infantile anxieties, and
- Tallness and psychological growth based on the containing functions of internal parents who perceive the Inner Child, experience the tears, anger, distress and joy of the Inner Child, and attempt to provide understanding and nurturance for this Inner Child.

I hold a different point of view from Dr Selvini Palazzoli's (1978) notion that anorectic young people are generally struggling for autonomy within their family. In my experience, young people with eating disorders are attempting to omnipotently evade their infantile emotions, which are part of the human experience of being intimately involved with other family members. Anorectics use omnipotent control, not autonomous functioning, which is based on identification with internalized caring parents who have a capacity for intimate relationships. Destructive omnipotent control against the conflicts of love and hate, which intimacy involves, needs to be differentiated from the capacity for autonomy, which is developed through maturely bearing and thinking about conflicting emotions.

The fear of being fat and of having too much food inside symbolizes the fear of being overwhelmed with infantile emotions without the proper internal parents to look after these emotions. Saying 'no' to food symbolizes the anorectic young person's need to 'say no' to the intense and difficult-to-bear good and bad experiences present in relationship to important people in their lives.

DOI: 10.4324/9781003044970-5

One anorectic girl described this very well when she said:

> I felt the toilet pipes were bursting. I also felt I was going crazy. I started knocking my head against the wall. Then I stopped eating, I turned away from others, my family and my friends. I fantasized stabbing my stomach when it was extended with food. I hated that fat!

For her there was a sense of cumulative traumatic, destructive experiences with limited intrapsychic structures to facilitate bearing bad internal or external experiences.

As I embarked on therapy with Riccardo and his family, I thought ideally, as the therapy progressed, Riccardo's wish to be tall would encapsulate his desire to have a psychic digestive system which could be 'grown-up', leaving him feeling 'tall' in identification with an internal father who was strong enough to have intimate relationships and experience loving and hating emotions, which he could digest and contain psychically.

The assessment phase

An anorectic child requires at least one individual assessment and two assessments with the entire family as well as a complete medical examination including weighing and charting a weight for height and age percentile. On the basis of this information, a decision regarding whether or not the child needs inpatient, outpatient or day treatment is made. Family therapy and/or couple counselling are felt to be essential and in combination with this, individual therapy is given to all children in the day treatment programme.

The individual assessment

In Chapter 2 I have outlined the way in which I involve the child in two individual assessments. I shall therefore simply show the assessment meeting with Riccardo in this chapter. My primary question is: 'What capacity does the individual, in identification with internal figures, have for looking after his own infantile self?' In empathically listening to a child and each family member, I hear the stories and tone of voice, as well as noting my emotional responses to the predominant attitudes present in his experiences, I then develop a picture of the current internalized parental figures and the infantile self. I also consider each individual's capacity to allow the internal parents to be together in various ways including for the procreation and care of the infantile self and siblings.

The nature of the internal parental figures will be influenced by the qualities of real parents and by the person's own feelings towards them. A stable sexual identity is sometimes based upon acknowledgment of one's gender, as well as identifying with both internalized parental figures performing their task of looking after the infantile self and joining together in creative ways. An individual's experience of his own body is influenced by these identifications with the internal parents and reflected in a sense of physical security and physical movements, as well as in the themes of the child's play, dreams and stories.

The first assessment session with Riccardo

Riccardo is a boy with three siblings: a brother, Emanuel, 16; a sister, Alma, aged six; and a sister, Carmella, aged four. When emaciated Riccardo came into the room I asked him to draw a picture for me. He drew a girl. He said that she lived with him and his sister. She had a relationship with her parents characterized by her shouting at them and then closing herself in her room. She was rather lonely in her room. I then talked with him about how the girl might be similar to him. He said that she was not similar in any way. I described the description he gave of her getting into an argument with her parents and then going away and staying alone in her room and when I wondered if that was something which he often did and he replied 'Yes, he did'. He quickly added, 'I like it that way.' I tried to explore what kind of pleasure he gained by being alone in his room. He said, 'It is not anything in particular that I like about being in my room, I simply like being alone.' He added, 'I don't like to do anything except work.' I wondered what particular kind of work interested him and he replied, 'Nothing in particular.' When I pressed him he said, 'Well, maybe history.' I asked about his history teacher and he said, 'He is excellent. You cannot really learn anything at school unless the teacher is someone you like, someone who is a good teacher like my history teacher.'

Then we talked about his current boarding school, which he had just left, and he said that he had not liked the previous school that he went to before he was nine, so his parents sent him to boarding school. The boarding school was where his brother Emanuel had been. Children entered this school after the age of 13. He liked the first two years there, but later on he did not like it at all because it was a very strict place. Riccardo indicated, 'The teachers actually beat the boys if they are not silent at night when it is their bedtime. I didn't get hit, but my friends did.' He commented that on the whole he liked to avoid that experience of being hit. He added, 'However, at times I did get in trouble for talking.'

When questioned, Riccardo responded, 'I am not happy at school, but I don't know why. I was surprised when I cried in the family meeting because I don't know why I would cry.' He was aware that other people in the family were sad, but he did not think it was true that the family did not communicate. I said, 'Perhaps the lack of communication that was being described was really about the tears which had not yet been put into words.' I added, 'Lack of communication might also refer to lack of communication between your achieving self and the unknown feelings within yourself.' Riccardo looked interested, but did not say anything in response to my comments.

Later, when I tried to explore the nature of his home life, Riccardo said, 'I like being friends with my brother [Emanuel, his 16-year-old brother]. I admire him and he is really good at playing the trumpet.' Spontaneously, Riccardo then added, 'About four years ago Emanuel frequently hit me for being a pest. I understood now why Emanuel did that for I was always trying to get his attention. Now that I am older I don't get hit by him and I like doing things with him.' Riccardo lamented, 'I don't see Emanuel much. He is always out, but I have another friend, called John, who lives nearby and we meet up quite often.' Riccardo said, 'At boarding school I know people, but I don't have any particular friends.' My impression was that Riccardo was quite isolated at his boarding school.

When I later tried to explore with Riccardo the pleasures he had in life, he seemed more alive as he replied, 'I like sports, any kind of sport: I like running and love wind-surfing. My dream is to wind-surf everywhere in the world once I get enough money.' He added, 'I go wind-surfing on the weekends with my dad. It's very exciting!' He also mentioned that he played the piano when he was at school, but he did not have his own horn in the inpatient unit and therefore did not play it now. Riccardo said, 'Even if I had the piano with me I would be embarrassed to make music which other inpatient children could hear'; however, he seemed rather interested in playing music if people could not hear him play.

When I inquired about his dreams, Riccardo replied, 'I sometimes have dreams, but somehow I have forgotten them now.' After a pause he mentioned, 'When I was six or seven I had frequent nightmares and often had difficulty sleeping. There were a lot of monsters in the dreams.' When I wondered how he responded to the nightmares, Riccardo said, 'I got into bed with my mother so I could try to sleep.' After further exploration with me, Riccardo remembered, 'I was often terrified by a red fiery dinosaur charging towards me.'

I also talked with Riccardo about whether he had been touched in any way that he would not like to be touched or in a way he felt was inappropriate. He indicated, 'No. I haven't been involved in any of that. I don't know any of the boys in school who were.' When I queried what he would do if something adverse happened to him, Riccardo said, 'Probably tell my parents.' He again mentioned, 'I haven't been hit by anyone except my brother, Emanuel.'

When I talked with Riccardo about how life could be made better for him, he described, 'I would like to do more things on the inpatient unit, I have to stay seated a lot of the time. Also, I enjoy school work, but the staff don't allow me to do any school work after school.' Vehemently he added, 'I don't like that one bit! I feel very claustrophobic just being inside the unit. I would like to go places and do things, that would really make life better for me.' I empathized with his feeling of being 'locked in', thinking to myself that he was also locked in by his obsessional anorectic thinking. I suggested that he could write down the kind of things he would like to do and together we could think more about this problem of being 'locked in' during our next meeting.

I subsequently talked more with him about this experience of withdrawing into his room or into himself and keeping away from people out of anger with them. I said,

> That there seems to be a pattern, a way of handling conflict, which you have and it is very easy to get stuck into that pattern of keeping to yourself. Now though we are trying to talk about what these conflicts are that concern you. This is one thing which we could try to understand more in therapy.

In reflecting upon his life, I sense that Riccardo has turned his loneliness into a position of feeling 'I like it this way'. This seems to be a defence against some of the pain of being lonely and alone. I say this because he does not really have anything behind this wall of isolation which gives him pleasure. He seems also to use work as a kind of 'wall' surrounding himself. Riccardo has more pleasure in his contact with peers than with adults. He is particularly keen on being involved with his brother Emanuel and his friend John.

Riccardo has not been able to sort out some of the resentment which he has towards his parents and school friends. There is no sense of his feeling nourished in any of his relationships with adult figures. They are portrayed mainly as disciplinarians who are somewhat distant from him, apart from the father with whom he enjoys wind-surfing. Also, Riccardo seems to have a healthy wish to have something better for himself, but he is very puzzled by an extreme hatred of having his body change from its present very thin, constricted shape. This may be linked both with anxieties both about maturing sexually and with his fear of his feelings getting out of control. He did mention, 'I get very worried when somebody feels that my voice indicates more anger than that of which I am aware.' It is for this reason that I feel Riccardo is worried about his feelings getting too big and transforming his personality from one which is governed by rational control into one which is out of control.

I continue to ask myself what makes this anorectic boy, Riccardo, different from an anorectic girl? He meets the same observable criteria for anorexia nervosa in girls. Present are:

- Determined food avoidance.
- Severe weight loss in the absence of illness.
- Preoccupation with body weight.
- Distorted body image.
- Fear of fatness.
- Extensive exercising.

He does not, however, abuse laxatives or vomit, as do some of the anorectic girls, particularly the older ones.

What interested me was that Riccardo was the only boy I have seen who, when asked to draw a human figure in the initial interview, drew a girl. I wondered if he had a fear of being identified with the 'roundness of his mother', the femaleness of his six-year-old sister, Alma, or the baby shape of his youngest four-year-old sister, Carmella. Certainly his fear of being fat with infantile feelings like his baby sister, and his fear of being feminine, might have influenced Riccardo's desire to control vigorously any hint of fat.

I have known five boys on the inpatient unit whose wish to avoid food concealed hypothalamic tumours. How could I differentiate Riccardo from these particular boys? Riccardo has a phobic fear of fatness and the pursuit of thinness. These particular feelings *must be present* to differentiate boys suffering from anorexia nervosa from boys with tumours leading to severe eating difficulties.

What I do know is that just as anorexia interferes with girls' body organs, brain cells, bones, teeth, hair, sexual development, including that of the ovaries, and long-term height, so also does it interfere with boys' physical and sexual maturity. Anorexia nervosa also lowers boys' sperm count with possible long-term consequences. Societal pressures rather than physiological causes are felt to be the primary reason that more girls than boys develop anorexia, but I suspect that it is also an identification with an ambivalent or hostile relationship with the mother that makes identifying with the mother's body damaged by hostility a source of feeling ugly, damaged and fat with disliked emotions. Also, of course, being sexually abused makes girls entering puberty fear getting pregnant and they may use anorexia nervosa as a contraceptive against both pubertal fears, the fear of getting pregnant and the anxieties regarding attracting undesirable males.

One year in our outpatient Eating Disorder Clinic for children seven to 15 years of age, 49 children were assessed and 11 of these (22%) of these children were boys. We have noted some potentially relevant factors in the development of eating disorders in males. These include the loss of family members, especially loss of males, learning problems, obsessive compulsive behaviour and the occurrence and impact of illness in infancy and early childhood (Lask and Bryant-Waugh, 1993).

Initial phases in family therapy

At times it is difficult to consider family therapy when research (Beresin, Gordon and Herzog, 1989) suggest that while half of one group of anorectic young people found family relationships to be a cause of their illness they found the family's attempt to help them to be harmful. In fact, over half of the anorectic young people felt that being away from the family was extremely helpful because of the family's hostile and derogatory remarks about not eating, the family's inability to understand the meaning of the illness, the lack of time to be involved with the anorectic child and feeling overwhelmed with the task of helping the child eat and not exercise or vomit.

One of the more successful British treatment centres, Rhodes Farm in London, separates the children from their families for a number of weeks, encourages the peer group to work together towards helping each other maintain a weight gain of 1 kilogram per week, while providing a combination of family therapy and individual therapy. At the Great Ormond Street Hospital, we do not separate the children from their families. Even if they are inpatients, the children see their families three times during the week. Generally on the weekends they go home if they can maintain their weight at home. We do, however, follow the model of individual and family work as well as having a parents' group and children's activity group on our inpatient and day programme for anorectic children.

I shall now describe four of the initial phases of therapy, illustrating my ways of understanding and working with the family of the anorectic boy, Riccardo, aged 12.

The Withdrawn Inner Child

As mentioned previously, the family consists of Emanuel, 16, Riccardo, 12 (the identified patient), Alma, six, and Carmella, four, father, a constrained and nervous tall, successful Italian stockbroker, and mother, who has a very intense, piercing look, wears glasses and dresses in a very plain, school-marmish way. She has concealed her emotional sensitivity with a very controlled, rather flat sounding voice. Mother is a university lecturer specializing in international relations and studying for a PhD.

In the first family session, mother introduces the family members and speaks about her son. Riccardo's anorexia has gone unnoticed for a long time, perhaps because he has done impressive academic work, to the point of perfection, and has a good relationship with his teachers. Riccardo was admitted to the inpatient unit because he was 70% weight for height and the hospital consultant psychiatrist noticed that Riccardo had gangrenous toes due to poor circulation. No one, including the family doctor, had previously seen his gangrenous toes!

The family interaction in the early sessions revealed the presence of a Withdrawn Inner Child present within most family members. The exception to this was the youngest girl, Carmella, four, who frequently ran for comfort, like a much younger child, to her mother or father's lap. As I contemplated the family interaction I assumed that in a healthy family, distress would be alleviated or modulated by the parental figures before the tension became intolerable. I felt that the Inner Child in all the older family members had been exposed to repeated and prolonged experiences of frustration. The children and parents' internalized parental figures seemed to be rather unreceptive to family members' emotions, which I am referring to as the Inner Child.

The way in which the Inner Child has attempted to cope with this situation of the inadequate support from internal and external parental figures has been to avoid contact with the external parental figures through every method available. The children rarely looked towards their parents. The family members rarely smiled or looked fondly at one another. When distressed no one, except Carmella, aged four, turned towards a parent for comfort. Where there were opportunities to share deeper feelings there seemed to be avoidance of emotionally laden encounters.

In one early family meeting I was particularly struck by Riccardo's avoidance of looking into his mother's eyes. When I mentioned this, Riccardo quietly retorted, 'I can hear my mother when she speaks, but I do not want to look into her eyes.' Mother later mentioned, 'My husband temporarily left me when Riccardo was one year old. During his absence I wanted nothing to do with Riccardo, because he reminded me so much of my husband who had hit me.' She also indicated, 'I have always felt intensely ambivalent towards both Riccardo and my husband.' Right after mother's comment, however, both mother and father described how Riccardo seemed the child in the family most similar to mother. Mother explained, 'This is because as a child I, like Riccardo, was depressed and had been prone to withdraw from my depressed mother.'

Ideally parental figures are nurturing, responsive and need-gratifying, but in turning to a depressed or hostile or unreceptive parental figure all that one would face is pain and rejection. The occurrence of intolerable disappointment in the parental figures resulted in a cut-off mechanism. This cut-off mechanism obliterated the experience of intolerable pain and disappointment in relationships with parental figures by getting rid of any awareness of needing parental figures or a marital partner, in the case of the parents. Emotional deprivation stemming from the lack of a supportive dialogue between the Inner Child and Parental Figures led to a transgenerational atmosphere of depression within the family.

Quote from sixth week of family therapy

The family is talking about Riccardo spending his first weekend at home. We are talking about pleasurable experiences, which the family could share over the weekend. Riccardo says, 'I don't want to do anything with my father.' 'Might you explain why?' I query. Riccardo keeps his head down and says nothing. Then he starts crying and says, 'I just want to keep to myself.' I suggest, 'It could feel safe, but lonely, in this way.' I then position a small child's chair next to Riccardo and I ask father to sit on it and speak to his son. Sitting in this chair, father matter-of-factly asks, 'Do you feel rather alone?' Riccardo looks at me and plaintively says, 'I don't want to be with my parents.'

Father asks him, 'What do you want me to do?' but he receives no response. After a pause I ask father to respond 'as Riccardo' to me and I ask, 'Why might you be crying?' In the role of Riccardo, father changes from being rather cold and intellectual to being quiet and plaintive as he replies, 'I want to be understood. All the time I am wanting more time together with the family.'

I then ask the 16-year-old son, Emanuel, to sit in the small chair 'as Riccardo'. 'What are you worried about?' I ask. Replying as Riccardo, Emanuel says, 'I am worried about my parents not trusting me about the weight.' From looking very complacent, Emanuel's expression changes to emanating concern. I try to move from the concrete discussion about food and weight and ask, 'Does your mother know why you are sad?' Emanuel, in the role of Riccardo, replies, 'Everyone in the family is probably sad.'

At this point mother starts crying and wiping away her tears. I gently request, 'Try to stay with the tears.' Mother blurts out to Riccardo, 'Your anorexia is a reflection of sadness in the family.' Father immediately bursts into the conversation, saying, 'The family has been sad since last summer.' Emanuel immediately adds, 'You are shutting yourself away from the family.' Riccardo defensively retorts, 'I don't want to think about the problems.' Father now returns to himself saying, 'No one is interested in what I am feeling. No one cares about what I am feeling'. At the end of the session, Carmella is sitting under her father's chair. She seems frightened by what is happening in the family.

The Inner Child turns to substitute objects

In his book, *Attachment and Loss*, Dr John Bowlby (1969) describes attachment behaviour as a tie that binds one person to another. It includes approaching, following and clinging to the object. The intensity of the attachment may be heightened or diminished by situational conditions. The pain of disappointing attachments to parental figures may contribute to the Inner Child attaching itself to 'false objects'. The more painful the disappointment with primary figures, the more intense the attachment to 'false objects' can become.

In this family, mother, father, Emmanuel, 16, and Riccardo, 12, Alma, six, Carmella, four, lacked an inner psychic structure to contain the painful disappointments in their relationships with each other. In this situation, these family members moved to a position of 'pseudo self-sufficiency' based on attachment to 'false objects. Work, academic studies, sports and music, activities which are usually signs of mature psychosocial adjustment, were turned to as means as 'omnipotent' methods of meeting these family members' need for human satisfaction. Alongside these potentially healthy activities, the older boy, Emanuel, also turned to drugs. All these activities had become means of turning away from primary needs for intimate relationships with people upon whom they could depend and with whom they could find love and pleasure. As a reflection of the family's general pattern, Riccardo's zealous studying to become a straight A student reflected not simply his interest in learning, but also his addiction to working to obtain 'top marks' both as a way of gaining the teacher's appreciation for his achievements and as a method of pushing away his dissatisfaction with human relationships.

In a subsequent family therapy session, mother complained, 'I am unhappy about my work being disrupted by Riccardo's anorexia requiring me spend time traveling to visit him in hospital.' I pondered aloud, 'How very difficult and complicated her life as a mother and wife was at home, with work, her university studies and Riccardo's anorexia.' Mother said, 'I might just disintegrate or lose my job if I miss work to come to a family therapy session.' During this conversation, Carmella, the four-year-old daughter, had drawn what she said was 'a picture of my mother leaving the house for work'.

Before Riccardo's emaciated anorectic body and gangrenous toes became visible to the family, to themselves and the outside world, the family felt themselves to be a normally functioning family. Only through the family sessions did it become apparent that the omnipotent destructive part of the personality (Rosenfeld, 1987a) had utilized healthy activities to attack potentially loving, caring and interdependent relationships with family and friends. Riccardo's non-stop sport activities and studying, Emmanuel's obsessive trumpet playing, Alma and mother's studying which completely obliterated the use of a dining room space for meals and father's excessive wind-surfing were used to blot out and attack any wish, on the parts of the Inner Child, to experience a need for intimacy with another person. These activities, which appeared so healthy on the surface, also enabled family members to devalue, attack and destroy, with pleasure, any wish of the Inner Child in each of them to depend on another person in the family. These potentially healthy activities were being used destructively to replace human intimacy.

The Inner Child voices a volcanic rage

My experience in doing observations of infants in the family and my work as a family therapist has led me to understand that the parents cannot help the Inner Child in their own children until the parents are able to listen to the Inner Child within themselves and receive some support from their partner and/or the therapist in bearing the Inner Child's intense emotions of love, possessiveness, hate and distress. I do not aim to primarily address marital conflict before helping the parents understand their children's feelings, but I do aim to give the parents some time both apart from and in front of the children to find ways of listening more attentively to the emotional meaning of the other's statements and to more deeply understand and identify with each other's Inner Child.

As part of the first four months of family therapy, I invite Riccardo's parents to have some regular sessions as a couple without the four children. In a quiet and receptive mood, I attempt to allow the couple to spontaneously bring any concerns which they wish to voice without the children present. With as little interference as possible by the therapist, what emerges from their unconscious interaction is a picture of the parents' shared internal parent figures and their Inner Child's relationship with these shared internal parent figures (Tereul, 1966).

In this couple the initial Shared Internal Parental Figure appears to be depressed, defended, unconcerned about the need for a dependable and understanding parent figure and often unaware of emotional distress and loneliness. This Shared Internal Parental Figure is a hardened, omnipotent structure which hides the Inner Child's volcanic hurt and rage.

What happens when there is a temporary relinquishment of the self-protective omnipotent, hardened 'super-parent' structure is that the couple experience panic. The panic is linked with the denied feelings which now emerge from the Inner Child. The unheard Inner Child appears feeling cruelly neglected and deprived by the lack of an understanding partner and the absence of a concerned internal parent. A volcanic rage about unmet needs emerges from the Inner Child. What is feared then is a violent rupture of the marriage. The presence of the therapist receiving the rage, gathering some if it into the transference, allows some security in voicing that which is unspeakable. The couple is encouraged to see how their unmet needs arise from previous parenting experiences, from their own and the therapist's inadequate listening to their own Inner Child, as well as because of their marital partner's inability to be responsive to their needs.

Here is an example of the Inner Child emerging in the third month of family therapy. Father says to his wife, 'You don't listen to my feelings. You just talk down to me. I don't like the tone of your voice.' Mother says, 'You ignore what I feel.' Father responds, 'I can't even tell what you are feeling, you are so rational when you speak, so unemotional.'

In helping the parents listen to their own unheard, abandoned and desperately needy, enraged Inner Child, and through assisting them to listen empathically to the Inner Child in the spouse, the couple become able to experience a genuine and increased concern from their own Inner Child and the spouse's Inner Child.

The following is an example from a subsequent session continuing the dialogue with the raging child. Father says, 'I've had 15 years of marriage. I want a lovely, happy life. I want to be with someone who loves me and whom I love.' Mother says, 'I do love you.' Father retorts, 'What you say and what you do are different.' Speaking furiously with a dramatic sweep of his arms to illustrate his point, Father goes on to say, 'I feel like I'm a teddy bear that is hugged every night and then thrown down in the morning and forgotten about.' In response, I describe the volcanic rage about unmet needs that has been held inside. Father says to mother, 'You stay all evening hidden in the dining room. You take over the entire room with books and paper. I can't even get you to tidy the mess so that at least I can do some work in the dining room.'

Mother then defensively complains, 'I have been feeling very unhappy and angry too.' Then, turning towards me she described, 'At that earlier time in my marriage my husband had hit me and bullied me, thus subduing me.' Looking towards her husband she firmly stated, 'Now I feel I have to be on top! I am determined to win each argument!' Rather triumphantly she remarks to me, 'It would be absolutely terrible to lose an argument with him [her husband]. Losing an argument would feel like having my identity crushed once again.' As mother speaks, I am reminded of Riccardo's holding onto his anorectic battle against his parents, unable to 'give in' to their wish for him to do eat normally, for fear that his anorectic identity, his omnipotent self would be crushed.

In response to the couple's outpouring of rage, I describe how the couple hold onto their emotional battles from the past. They felt they HAD TO BE forceful and strong, with father holding onto long hours at work and mother focused mainly on her books and papers, which transform the dining room into an office.

In the next session, as the parents continue their complaints, I ask them to sit in the centre of the room with their backs touching each other. I describe the wall of long hours of work and also quietly describe. 'The nurturing spaces are all filled with stacks of work papers.' I delineate this 'wall of work' depicted by their backs barricading each of them from the other. Gently I ask each of them separately to tell their partner how they feel behind the 'wall of work'.

Father quickly responds, 'I am very worried about my wife working very hard, getting an even better job through her studies and then leaving the marriage.' He adds, 'I feel she is selfish when she won't perform her motherly duties and agree to fetch the younger children from their school activities and visit Riccardo in hospital on Monday mornings.' Mournfully he continues, 'I need to keep up with the fast pace of my business which I don't enjoy, but my wife wants to go to her university lecturing job and study all the time.' Mother adamantly replies, 'Saying yes to my husband means giving into his selfishness.' Father confesses, 'I am so angry with her that I can't compromise.' Mother quietly responds, 'I feel the same way.'

I empathically describe the strong wall of anger between them. Then I suggest,

> You both seem to have a 'shared internal figure', a hard figure, an unnurturing figure, a figure that can't make any concessions. Hearing the emotional needs of the other is viewed as submitting, being weak, surrendering to an uncaring, selfish figure. Each partner complains that the other can't hear the others needs or respond to each other's wishes.

Then mother remembers, 'I continually wanted to get my emotionally distant father's approval through working hard and impressing him through my academic achievement. Only my father simply remained distant and didn't really pay any attention to me even when I tried to be loving to him.' Father tells a similar story about his relationship with his mother. Shortly afterwards I ask the parents to face one another. Speaking softly and tenderly to the Inner Child in each of them I say, 'Each of you is longing to be comforted, needing to be understood and each of you has been terribly disappointed and starved of caring by a loving parent.' I go on to show, in various detailed ways, how the Inner Child had been terribly disappointed in human relationships *before* they came together as a couple and also now. I illustrate this by saying, 'In your separate ways, you avoid the terrible pain of being hurt and neglected by "holding on for dear life" to your work. Your work has become the source of security.' I continue by saying, 'The problem is that the little Inner Child cannot be properly nourished and comforted through attaching itself to work. It can only be nurtured and properly understood through the intimacy of a relationship with oneself and one another.' I proceed by illustrating, 'You each married while sharing a hurt, but very sensitive Inner Child. You needed one another. You needed one another to repair the hurt inside.' Going further, I wonder, 'Now how can you help each other stay in touch with each other's heart? Is there a way?' At this point mother starts crying profusely. After a while she says, 'I hadn't realized before how desperately I was holding onto work for security and how I was barricading myself from my husband. No wonder I can't stop work to visit Riccardo; I need work for my security.' As she spoke father noticeably softened his 'hard shoulder' stance and his face showed that he was very moved by his wife's tears and words.

Again, I wonder aloud, 'Are there any ways in which the Inner Child might find another source of security besides work?' The parents' body postures suggest more vulnerability as the session draws to a close.

Building a home for the Inner Child

When the parents return, with all four children, for the next family session the couple seem closer emotionally and more sensitive as they speak. I wondered if expressing pent-up hurt and hostility freed them to be more emotionally connected. They start talking about how Riccardo was feeling uncomfortable and trapped in the hospital ward. Since Riccardo was not speaking in response, I suggested that Emanuel, his 16-year-old brother, sit beside him to describe what he felt Riccardo might be feeling, as well as what he himself was feeling. Just before he spoke I encouraged the parents to simply listen attentively to whatever the boys had to say. As I listened I became increasingly aware of how the parents' capacity to support each other and acknowledge their own sadness had transformed them somehow in Riccardo's eyes. I experience this as I hear Riccardo, for the first time, speaking to his parents about his unhappiness. He starts crying as he tells them what he had never been able to tell them before: 'The entire previous year in boarding school I have been unhappy.' When questioned by his mother he painfully mumbles, 'Other boys receive letters from their parents and I don't. Other parents call their sons two or three times a week, but you rarely call me.'

Remarkably, as though reflecting a new more benign internal state of the family, during this discussion Carmella, aged four, is drawing a house. Meanwhile, Alma, the six-year-old, is gathering bricks, unloading them and beginning to build a house near her father's chair. I felt their play reflected a new possibility for all the family members. It seemed the family was developing a kind of emotionally containing cradle involving receiving projections, unwanted feelings and intense desires of each family member's Inner Child. Having experienced my emotional support and having disclosed some of their hurt and hostility, the parents now seem potentially receptive enough to provide 'a house' for their children's feelings. Riccardo, on behalf of his siblings, somehow feels this and is expressing his hurt and anger towards the parents.

Letting go of omnipotent control to discover a home for the heart

Once the parents reveal hints of being able to transform 'the internal hard super-parent omnipotent structure', there emerges the possibility of new areas of feeling and thinking. Riccardo's sadness is now openly present. He is momentarily released from his imprisoning anorectic stance of staying in his room, studying and starving, while appearing to want no one. Now, for the first time in his life, when his parents are more supportive to one another and feel 'less hard', Riccardo gives way to outbursts of hurt and anger about all sorts of things. Firstly he becomes furious with his key worker, a male nurse on the unit who was away for a two-week leave of absence. Then in the session, Riccardo angrily tells his mother she is *over* anxious, overprotective and treating him like a younger child, not a 12 year old. At the same time, Riccardo remains riddled with anorectic body sensations, saying, 'I just feel too "well-rounded". I don't like that feeling. I just want to be tall.'

After Riccardo angrily complains to his mother, I suggest,

> 'the family home' is overflowing with so many feelings of the 'Inner Child' hidden away for so long by all the family's achievement-oriented activities. Riccardo is speaking for the family, showing his vulnerability, his sad feelings, his wish to be close, but not too close to people in his family.

I suggest, 'No one wants simply to be at the mercy of these angry, painful, intense feelings of the Inner Child.' However, I am able to add,

> Now something different is being experienced by each of you. You see the potentialities of having someone in your family who will really listen to you. There is a sense of there being a mother, a father, parents ready to be present for the 'Inner Child'.

I talk also of the recently revived feelings about father being 'a courageous man' when he was involved in an Italian military rescue mission. I add, 'Now you have a choice – to find "a home for each other in your heart" or to continue to barricade yourselves with a wall of work.'

This is just the first four months of family therapy. In the next one and a half years, including time when Riccardo returned home, family therapy continued. Riccardo went to a new non-residential school near his home and began starving again. Alongside the family therapy I provided telephone counselling at regular fixed intervals, initially daily, to enable the parents to successfully assist Riccardo with his eating difficulties in order that he could remain home rather than going into hospital again. Gradually he settled into his new school.

Follow-up report

Two years after family therapy ended, Riccardo had some friends whom he saw regularly. He was 100% weight/height and he was developing sexually. Riccardo, having grown 8 cm each year, was also pleased to note that he 'would be tall', rather than stunted in his growth. At the end of treatment, we always give the family a written form as well as a session to evaluate what has taken place during the course of the treatment. Riccardo's family commented that initially they simply felt a deep shock about the severity of the problems. They felt the trauma itself necessitated changes in their ways of communicating. In conjunction with the therapy offered, they felt they 'had become more understanding of the children's needs'. Parental depression and ambivalence towards the children were cited as being more intense than could be acknowledged in the family sessions. In the later stages of therapy they had begun to work together as a family with more sensitivity to each other.

Theoretical discussion

My work with families of anorectic children is constructed on a psychoanalytic model. At the same time, I work in continual liaison with a medical doctor, preferably a child psychiatrist who initially and then fortnightly examines the physical condition of the child heart, blood, circulation, sexual development, dehydration, wasting level and the necessary presence of potassium and zinc.

Mobilizing external people to restore a healthy eating pattern

I also ensure that someone in the external environment, whether it be staff or family members, intervenes immediately in assisting the child to develop normal eating patterns. Early intervention in the eating pattern ensures the best long-term prognosis for the child. Research confirms that it is much better to ensure recovery from the disturbance of nutrition and eating in order to facilitate the anorectic young person's psychological health to work in insight-oriented therapy. The network of external helpers and the therapist attempt to take away starvation as the battleground so that other areas of potential family conflict can be explored. In London's Great Ormond Street Hospital we advocate that psychotherapists need to work in collaboration with medical doctors who know about ways of assessing and talking to anorectic young people. Individual psychotherapy works too slowly to help the severely ill child assume total responsibility for eating to restore normal bodily functions; hence it is *essential* that an individual psychotherapist involves a network of the necessary professionals to assist the family to help their child eat and continue letting go of their anorectic control as well as developing intimate relationships with family members. If the family cannot do this through outpatient treatment, nurses doing home-visiting or day treatment programmes involving the parents are the first treatments of choice. Sometimes, however, as in the case of Riccardo, the body is too unwell to risk the child remaining out of hospital.

Containment

Within the family sessions as well as in the regular telephone counselling sessions offered to caregivers of the child, and in work with the professional network caring for the family, the central burden on the family therapist is that of containing unbearable death and life anxieties. Also, the anxieties to do with possessiveness, greediness, the wish to control rather than bear emotions of love, desire and pain, give rise to conflictual and sometimes hostile and persecuting interactions between family members and between the network of professionals involved with the family. Unresolved conflicts between the parents, between the parents and the clinical team and within the professional group all impede the therapeutic progress of the family and the anorectic young person in the family. Containment of anxieties and reduction of hostile interactions is especially important for anorectic young people. Even the parents' low levels of criticism expressed towards the anorectic young person are associated with the continuation of anorectic symptoms (Le Grange et al., 1992). This seems to do with the blaming process based on a feeling of impotence leading to projection, splitting, self-hatred and denial. If these processes get underway, they are hard to overcome and can prevent family therapy from being an effective treatment for anorexia nervosa (Dare, 1993).

Noting current interactions of the Inner Child

The focus of the work is the transferences in the present moment of the family members' interactions. The here and now in the therapeutic setting is the meeting point of the past and the present family's unconscious internal dramas as it expresses itself. Primarily I am fostering the optimal conditions for each family member to hear their own Inner Child and listen carefully with understanding to what is being expressed. I also encourage the family members to experience and identify compassionately with the Inner Child of the other family members. Younger children are free to play spontaneously in the course of much of the session and I try to think with the family about the meaning of their free play.

Therapeutic style

I try to work in an enlivening and engaging way with the warmth and neutrality that comes through fostering identification with the Inner Child in each family member. This involves me in re-positioning my little chair next to different family members and encouraging them to move their chairs in order to have an important dialogue with a particular family member. For example, I might have one of the children move closer to face both parents or move the parents to face one another. Role-reversal with different children or the parents taking the place of a particularly quiet child in the family becomes a way of amplifying inadequately expressed feelings of one's own Inner Child. It also facilitates understanding through identification with the Inner Child in the other.

Nurturing

The family therapist's role is that of a nurturing figure who provides a setting where feelings can be looked at gradually in a way that can be tolerated by the family members. The family therapist provides an opportunity for the emergence of truthfulness in the dialogue between the Inner Child and the Internal Parents as well as between the Inner Child and the external parents. Hopefully this truthfulness can lend emotional nourishment and support the development of the internal figures of each member of the anorectic young person's family. Thus the family can 'grow tall' with maturity while restricting the 'fatness' of unbearable infantile feelings through digesting them through holding them and lending them thought.

Chapter 5

The eye turned inward

Hallucinations in severe eating disorders

At night we live our dreams, actively engaged in the dream activity, as though it were real. An adolescent with a severe eating disorder, however, may begin to move into the internal world in a waking state. She hears the voices of the internal world, views the images, sounds, smells and sensations of unconscious phantasies. At the same time, however, in therapy, the girl is maintaining an awake, day-time thoughtful self, describing her hallucinations to the therapist. I am still rather surprised when I receive an affirmation yes to these assessment questions:

- 'Is there a voice or someone around influencing you that no one else knows about?'
- 'Is it located outside you?'

In this chapter I shall discuss one of many ways of thinking about hallucinations in children, using my clinical work with adolescents who have eating difficulties. I shall use the word hallucination to define a false perception that is not a sensory distortion or misinterpretation of a physical form, sensation or sound, but occurs at the same time as though it were a real perception of an external reality. The hallucination is a sensory impression having a concrete reality and objectivity and when communication is possible the hallucination is defined in a clear and detailed manner as having a constancy independent of will.

There are hallucinations accompanying bereavement, which are felt to be normal for a period of time. There are also hallucinations linked with organic damage. Pseudo-hallucinations and eidetic imagery would be able to be distinguished as being seen inside the mind or known not to be real by the child. They are often ill-defined or images of deceased relatives. There is a hazy border or continuum of pathological features between hallucinations and pseudo-hallucinations in children who lack sufficient communication skills or the cognitive capacity to describe the hallucinations.

I am aware that the voice or figure that is being hallucinated can have many different helpful or detrimental roles in relation to the adolescent. I am

DOI: 10.4324/9781003044970-6

bearing in mind that Socrates and Joan of Arc heard voices. Probably 400 years ago, in the days when everyone seemed to believe in devils and angels, voices and apparitions were a much more common feature of society. Also in some cultures, such as the Philippines, it would be considered an ordinary experience for people to hallucinate deceased relatives for up to 40 days after their death.

I shall share with you some of my uncertainty and understanding about working therapeutically with eating disordered young people having hallucinations. The hallucinations of one girl, Helena, will be described, followed by a picture of how she was able to develop an inner dreaming space which enabled her to work with her anxieties regarding the hallucinations. I shall also allude to two other hallucinating girls, Caterina and Amelia.

In a traumatic experience, the young person experiences a state of helplessness. The Self fears disintegration, bombardment, fragmentation and has acute anxiety about how to manage the trauma. The trauma is due not only to whatever external precipitating event may be present, but also to the conjunction of this external trauma with the overwhelming anxiety that the internalized parents' ego functions will be destroyed. Ideally, at the time of an emotional disaster, the child will turn to parental figures, both within the Self and outside the Self, to attempt to take care of the self having a traumatic experience. The traumatizing feelings need to be recognized, experienced and emotionally understood. When the inner infantile Self cannot find the protection and understanding required from either the inner parental figures, the ego, and/or external parental figures, the Self requires some way of remaining psychically active. Fear of death of the Self brings the fear of actual physical death. Perhaps sometimes death through physical causes, like a heart attack, does occur at times when the Self cannot live.

From infancy onwards, there is an option available to save the Self from nameless dread and fear in the absence of a parental figure. This option is to hallucinate a figure and attach oneself to it. Sigmund Freud (1911, p. 119) describes the breast-feeding experience, which is dreamt about, or the feeding breast, which is hallucinated in the absence of the feeding mother. Research has indicated that these hallucinations bring about some physiological responses very similar to those when the breast is really present. For this reason, we can say that the hallucination does have some instinctive survival value for the suffering Self. The hallucination is turned to when there is a crisis of psychic survival.

Beside wish-fulfilling hallucinations there are also persecutory ones such as those of monsters. For example, some anorectic young people have fragile mothers who are unsupported by their husbands. In these instances, the young people consciously or unconsciously fear that showing hostility or disappointment to a very vulnerable external parent will result in the external parent becoming too hurt, too damaged, too persecuted or too filled with a destructive revenge towards the child. A similar situation in which hostility is not consciously acknowledged may occur when there is an internal harsh, punitive superego causing persecutory guilt.

At moments such as these, instead of confronting the external parents, the child may project her destructive feelings into an internalized mother or father figure. When there is too great an accretion of internal conflict and there is no way of containing it emotionally, the eye turns inward to internal parents or siblings which are often projected outside the Self. At times, though, these damaged internal figures can become concretized in the body, particularly in young children who imagine a little monster in their body. In adolescents, when there is too much internal conflict, the internal phantasy often becomes projected via the eyes or ears, or nose into an external hallucination. This projection from the body into external images, voices and sometimes accompanying smells represents an attempt to get out of the internal trauma in which the Self feels helpless. At the same time the child may retain an idealized external mother figure or therapist. Or at the very least, the child maintains a relationship with external parents and/or a therapist which seems free of conscious conflicts.

I have seen a group of fragile anorectic children who have developed hallucinations when they were in what I believe to be an unethical behavioural program requiring them to be isolated from family and friends until they ate the required number of calories and gained weight or when they were faced with sharp, sudden hospitalization, which involved periods of unbearable separation from their parents.

As time progresses, without therapy, the child may become preoccupied with her hallucinatory figures, turning her eye increasingly toward her inner world and projecting it outward into an hallucination. Because of their disturbing nature, or because of their novelty, the child may cling to the hallucinations like a teddy bear hugged in moments of distress. The child feels that the hallucinations may protect against suffering more effectively than anyone else. Hallucinations can become so attractive as to become addictive, like a drug that is used to obliterate the pain of external reality. In these instances, the hallucinatory figure can become so filled with parts of the Self that it can become more potent than the Self and dominate the Self. The hallucinatory experience is then felt to be a terrifying enemy of the sane part of the Self. It can attempt to rob the sane part of its sanity and take its place. In fact, the major aim of the insane part of the Self is to take over the relationship that the sane part has with reality and to dominate the sane part. As therapy progresses, the hallucinations can compete with the child's emotional dependence on the therapist. For example, a hallucinatory voice may utter destructive remarks such as, 'Don't listen to the therapist, if you do, I'll kill her.' These figures are against eating food, representing life, and against maintaining an intimate emotional link with important primary figures and/or the therapist.

I have seen or supervised the psychotherapy of five eating disordered young people who have lived for an extended period of time in the company of hallucinatory figures. These different types of hallucinatory figures have changed in quality and function as the young person developed more internal capacity for thinking about her emotions. I shall describe the experiences of three of these adolescent girls.

All three girls, Helena, Caterina and Amelia were inpatients when they began psychotherapy. Two, Caterina and Amelia, aged 14, were both suffering from what is classically known as anorexia nervosa. Their symptoms included food avoidance, the fear of fatness, a distorted body image; severe weight loss, over 25% of their normal body weight, making them below the 75% weight for height for their age and causing loss of their ordinary menstrual cycle. Helena, 14, upon whom I shall primarily focus, suffered from not eating, fear of fatness, but also she could not walk and did not talk at the time of admission. She could be described as having what we at Great Ormond Street Hospital called pervasive avoidance-withdrawal syndrome (PAWS) obscuring anorectic thinking.

Helena first arrived in the hospital curled up in a wheelchair. Very thin, with a spotty complexion, she persistently played with her long red hair, which she held in front of her eyes. Her difficulties had begun a year earlier when Helena developed an earache for which no physical cause could be found. She stayed home for several months until her parents took her to the paediatrician who encouraged them to send her back to school. Helena felt very unhappy about this plan and it later emerged that she felt her parents had not taken the extent of the physical pain seriously enough when they followed the paediatrician's advice. Having returned to school, Helena gradually stopped eating normally. Five months later she gave up walking completely. Later, when placed in the paediatric unit, separate from her parents with whom, at age 14, she still usually slept, she stopped talking.

Helena was then moved from the paediatric unit to the inpatient unit, which normally opens five days a week. She spent the weekends at home. On Mondays, when her mother said goodbye to her, Helena began a violent, loud, desperate cry which regularly lasted for up to three hours. She would simultaneously bang her head against the wall and punch her own eyes. She also picked the skin off her lips until they bled and scratched her face. The nurses would have to physically restrain her for hours. As she calmed down, Helena began fiddling with her long red hair, twisting it round her fingers, holding it in front of her eyes, staring at it. When she later uttered words they blurred into indistinguishable chants. We sensed that they were repetitious phrases.

Helena's crying was intolerable to the therapeutic care workers as well as to her mother. Mother actually cried for at least several days after leaving Helena in the unit on Mondays because she could not bear Helena suffering while being separate from her. After three months the staff felt quite desperate about Helena's continuous chanting and piercing cries which occurred each time she was separated from her parents. For this reason they arranged for me to see Helena and asked that I be present at that precise moment when her mother left her in hospital. I agreed to work with Helena but suggested that I work together with Helena and both parents with regard to the separation until she could separate from them. Subsequently, I began seeing Helena in individual therapy sessions, which felt more like an infant observation in which I was verbalizing what I observed and experienced in witnessing Helena's non-verbal communication and her parents' responses to her. I was attempting to enable the parents to find a way of greeting and understanding the inner child in Helena. Using my countertransference responses, I took into consideration her body posture, glances and position, stillness or movement of her fingers, hands or legs. This was not the family therapy, which was being done by another psychotherapist on a fortnightly basis. I also saw Helena once a week without her parents.

Over time Helena began to tell her mother at home what I should know about her. For example, she told her mother to tell me that she cried when the doctor said she must go back to school. When her mother told me this in the session, I dramatized that scene in front of Helena and her parents. Simultaneously I used the dolls to hold Helena's visual attention, since she often seemed to have lost the capacity for listening to words. Holding a male doll, I spoke for the doctor, saying, 'There is nothing wrong with her ear. You should send her back to school.' Then I held a small girl doll saying to two parent dolls, 'But nobody understands that I am in pain. I am suffering.' I then spoke directly to the Helena doll, saying, 'I wonder if you feel that no one understood how you felt inside. Perhaps you felt rejected by everyone and perhaps furious that no one understood how you felt.' At this point Helena began to weep copiously.

Gradually, at home, Helena began asking her mother to tell me about her pain. In the session, mother would then describe 'the pain' to me. Helena had said that the pain was that she had no memory of the past. She did not remember or recognize the cat, the house, her younger sister, or her school friends. From the teacher I learnt that Helena had lost her memory of the alphabet and numbers and could not concentrate, read or do maths. She also did not draw.

Subsequently, Helena indicated that the pain occurred when she separated from her mother. At that moment she had visions of her mother crying for her and of visions of her mother dead. These hallucinations were extremely frequent when her mother was away from her, initially filling many of Helena's days in hospital. Upon questioning, I learned that the hallucinations occurred very quickly after mother departed. Slowly the nurses and I deciphered Helena's chanting, which occurred when mother left her. The chant included the phrase, 'Please don't hurt my mum' and 'I love you, mum.' The hallucination and accompanying chanting occurred simultaneously with Helena fiercely hitting her eyes and scratching her face. I sensed that in hitting herself, Helena was attacking her internal mother, the departing mother. She was psychically parasitically residing as a baby inside this mother. In her simultaneous chanting Helena was attempting to protect this loved mother from her hitting that was taking place.

A few weeks after she had begun therapy, Helena said to her mother that she had found a little man in her hand whom she watched while he spoke to her. Nine months after her earache commenced, she had begun speaking to him two or three times a day. Slowly Helena revealed what happened in her relationship with this 'little man' in her hand. At night, alone in the hospital bedroom, there was no longer a little man in her hand. Over time he had developed into a big man who appeared on the wall. At times he looked like her father's much-loved older brother who had died two years before. He gave her messages during her weekends at home. He also spoke to her while she was in the hospital. I felt it was essential to become acquainted with this hallucinated uncle and to explore with Helena the nature of her relationship with him.

It seemed important that I treat this man with respect and get to know him, rather than attempting to destroy this hallucination, to which she was desperately clinging. Interestingly, as the work proceeded, it emerged that Helena was no longer turning to him as before. Instead he beckoned her, forced himself into the focus of her attention and told her what to do. I assumed that the man grew more powerful as Helena split off and projected more parts of her personality into him. When she became more dependent on sharing her emotional experiences with me she became emotionally healthier. When the hallucinated man became larger, Helena was tyrannized by him. Helena said that 'the big man' told her, 'Do not follow the advice of the nurses on the unit! Do not eat! Do not get better!' He also threatened Helena, saying, 'You should not get better, for if you do, your mother will die.'

Despite the hallucinatory figure's threats, Helena continued to tell her mother what to reveal to me in the session. She described how, when she had had this earache, other things happened as well and they still continued. Mother came into the bathroom because Helena could not walk alone. Helena indicated, 'When you leave the bathroom, I look down into the bath-tub and see all sorts of bodies with blood oozing out of them.' Helena added, 'Sometimes, when alone at night, I look up at the bedroom ceiling and see skeletons with skulls and no flesh. This terrifies me.'

Helena was still not speaking to me in the sessions. In the silence I used the dolls to dramatize the stories she had told her mother to tell to me. The dolls seem to hold her attention, whereas she simply drifted away from my undra-matized ordinary verbal communication. Week by week I held a small doll and facing the doll I talked about the 'little Helena's experiences'. I closely observed Helena's reactions as I talked to the doll and I tried to understand my emotional experience of being with her. For example, I would describe, 'You seem to feel better with me when your mother is with us. It feels safe then. When you are alone in the bedroom, without mother, without me, you become frightened of those skeletons on the ceiling.' I described the skeletons. I talked, looking at the Helena doll, about 'little Helena': 'You feel you cannot be alone, you *should not* be alone. All these terrible visions occurred when you are alone. You are terrified of these visions and need to be with mother, to be with me, to feel safe.'

Helena seemed to be interested when I told these stories, facing the 'Helena doll', or identified with the Helena doll listening to the hallucinated man, or I spoke with the hallucinated man doll's voice. I slowly showed the Helena doll, feeling furious to be left alone. Everyone turned bad and she then turned to the man on the wall. Then the hallucinated man would speak. Only gradually did I share my thoughts about what the dolls were feeling and how this related directly to Helena. I felt she firstly needed to think about experiences located in a space apart from her on the table where I put the dolls, where I put the feelings in a doll *outside her mind*. Subsequently I began to describe how 'little Helena' was terrified alone without mother or me. I would show the doll hitting herself, peeling the skin off her lips, feeling torn apart from mother. I also talked about the rage of 'little Helena' towards mother departing, towards me departing.

Just at this point Helena, interrupted me and spoke for the first time! Speaking directly to me she said firmly, 'No, I'm not angry.' She would listen to my comments about her terror of separation and her fear that no good mother was alive. However, she could not listen to any stories I told about 'little Helena' being very hurt and cross with the mother or me going away or Helena hurting mother, or hitting 'mother inside', represented by Helena's punching of her own eyes. Consciously Helena felt attacked and abandoned by mother at the point of separation. She was not ready to tolerate any other thoughts about her experience of being torn away from mother. For this reason, Helena adamantly continued to disagree with me when I talked about her anger or crossness. I felt she was correcting me in a helpful way. She still felt resident inside mother and undifferentiated from the mother who was in Helena's phantasy hurt and damaged by the separation. Moreover, Helena had been denying these feelings of rage towards her mother for 14 years, protecting her depressed mother from these feelings. I had been prematurely asking her to become conscious of rage. This was impossible. Her experience was that she psychologically fell apart when mother left. Her world turned into terrifying, bloodied people.

However, as far as I was concerned, Helena's disagreement with me represented a development for it reflected her sense that I could bear her being in conflict with me. I went on using the dolls, talking about 'little Helena' wanting mummy all the time, 'little Helena' not wanting mummy and I to talk together. Each time I mentioned emotions which appeared hostile, Helena would say firmly, 'I'm not jealous. I don't want my mother all the time.' She would not agree to any descriptions of negative emotions such as anger, rage, jealousy or possessiveness. Hostility to the primary figure, mother, me, could not yet be consciously thought about by Helena.

I understood that the chanting with visions of mother being killed linked with an internal figure who was not only fragile, damaged and unable to bear intense pain of separation. The mother was conceivably unconsciously attacked by Helena. 'I love you, mum', the second phrase of the chant, reflected Helena's wish not to hurt mother through her infantile rage. One problem was that neither Helena nor her mother could tolerate or distinguish between the pain of separation and the experience of an absolute tragedy. Both cried for hours when separated. Separation felt like a tearing apart, an endless trauma or death.

As has been the case with the five hallucinating girls I've seen, the feared internal tragedy is not only linked with jealous, possessive and hostile emotions directed to the parental couple. Helena's internal situation was complicated by the fact that Helena had actually prevented her father, who was often visibly restraining his internal explosiveness, from hitting her mother on one occasion. Also after her father had shouted in a fierce and frightening way at her uncle, her beloved uncle had died. It seemed as though in Helena's mind, expressing emotions of anger and rage seemed to be equated with physically hurting or killing someone. She dis-identified with her father, perhaps projecting her rage into him.

This became clear in one of the later sessions when, after in a therapy session, Helena spoke directly to her father. She asked her father, 'Why did you yell at my uncle?' (This was the much-loved uncle who had died.) I suggested Helena say more about why she was asking. Helena replied, 'My father made my uncle die.' She then corrected herself, saying, 'He made him die sooner.' She added, 'My uncle had blood coming out of his mouth.' (He had had a haemorrhage.) Afterwards I talked to Helena, saying,

> You feel that anger kills. How difficult it is to imagine anger being a feeling in one's head? It is possible to share a feeling of anger inside one's head by talking rather than shouting. If someone is able to listen, anger can be safely shared by talking.

I added, 'Rage can have a limit, a place to stop.'

Helena then courageously and complainingly said to her father:

> Why are you horrible to me? Why do you tell me to walk? I will walk when I feel happy! I'm not happy now. I'm not going to walk now. I just want to die when you and mum try and make me walk or eat.

Helena did not want anyone to interfere with her psychic retreat to non-stop residence 'inside mother's womb' before she was ready.

Helena's partial residence in a hallucinatory world was being threatened by her continuing dialogue with me. As she became more dependent and conversant with me, she told me, 'When I am with you the voices are getting louder, I can barely hear you.' She wouldn't tell me what 'the big man' and the other voices said. She told me, 'You will get angry with them if you know what they say!' It seemed that as she reached towards life, the anxiety regarding change in her psychic equilibrium produced a competition between 'the voices' and me. The voices were part of herself, clung to as part of her 'protection service', and they were being threatened by my presence. Helena began to reveal, 'The voices are threatening me that they will only go away if I hurt myself.' They are saying, 'If you do not scratch yourself right then in the session, then we will make you use a knife to cut yourself later.' In fact, as Helena began to emerge from her hallucinatory cocoon, she began scratching her wrists with various objects. Her wish for life was being attacked. Physical hurt seemed better than emotional suffering connected with loss of the hallucinations, loss of mother, and knowing about her own greedy impulses, her own fears. But now, Helena was able to talk with me about the attacks on her life. It was clear, mother was not allowed to be separate from Helena. Also, though, according to these threatening voices, Helena was not allowed to eat, to walk and thus exist outside this imprisoning internal mother in whom she had been psychologically residing.

Through some work in family therapy, the parents had decided to go out together for the first time in over a year. When they told Helena of their evening out in the session, Helena calmly threatened, 'If you leave me I will throw myself out of the window. I will also kill my babysitter.' She fiercely insisted, 'If you go out together I will never get better. I will kill myself.' Now Helena's terror of separation, her violent rage about separation from her mother and her oedipal jealousy of the couple having pleasure together was out in the open. Also, Helena had now consciously begun to own some of her previously unconscious split off hostility towards me. This was obvious as she disagreed more openly with me in the sessions rather than telling me 'the voices' were saying terrible things about me.

Unfortunately I was away for an unexpectedly long period. At this point Helena asked the unit if she could meet with her keyworker every day. The staff were extremely surprised by Helena's request, since at that time she was barely speaking to the nurses, but they agreed to her request. In Helena's wish to meet her keyworker in daily meetings, I felt Helena was indicating that there had been a significant change in her capacity to face the reality of separation from someone important to her. An understanding therapist with whom one could share worries had been preserved inside her, even though I was away. The sharp reality of my sudden departure alongside the presence of daily sessions with her capable keyworker nurse contributed to a fundamental shift in Helena's psychological structure for facing crises. Previously in facing separation Helena had entered the world of her auditory and visual hallucinations. Now she was using her awareness of an internalized supportive therapist to ask for help from her keyworker. Helena was also able to sufficiently contain distressing emotions about separation to be able to dream, remember her dreams and take an interest in them.

The keyworker enabled Helena to discuss some of her predominating worries and dreams in the last ten weeks of her hospital admission.

This is the first dream:

> I am shopping looking at 'a lot of things to make things' on the shelves. Many people are in the shop. I go back to my uncle's house. I sit on his lap, while my mum and dad are sitting together in the other chairs. I look under my uncle's shirt and see there is nothing there from the waist to the neck but a T-shirt. I realize that he has been that way the whole time. He's dead. I start screaming and run out of the house. Mum and dad are sitting there normally.

(Note: Since her illness, Helena had lost much of her capacity to name many objects and could only describe their functions or visual features. If she had been able to find the words about what was on the shelves she would have been talking about flour, milk, vegetables and other food in the supermarket.)

In the second dream, Helena describes:

> I am at the home of my aunt and uncle. They are all having dinner together and everyone is eating. I am talking to my aunt and uncle. When my mother and father walk in they ask me who I am talking to. Dad says, 'Nobody is there.' When I look there is nothing there. My aunt and uncle have gone. My mother and father say that I have been eating the aunt and uncle for dinner. I start crying and screaming. I run away. My mum and dad are smiling.

In describing the third dream, Helena says:

> My uncle is not alive. He is dead, but he looks just the same as when he was alive. I run to a friend's house for safety. When I come out of the house, my uncle starts chasing me again. My parents shout for me to come back but I am afraid that they may be cross. A lady is going past in her car. I jump in her car and ask for help. When I get out, my parents, my sister and my uncle start chasing me.

In communicating her fourth dream, Helena says:

> I am sitting in the sitting room on my own. My uncle knocks on the door. I answer the door. I see my uncle who is a skeleton. He asks for something to eat. I say, no, because I don't like him. My uncle falls into a pile of bones when I say no. Everybody hates me because they think that I have killed my uncle.

These dreams are terrifying. They express the verdict, 'The uncle is dead.' They also suggest that Helena knows that she can easily turn to the hallucinated uncle figure when she is in a room alone thinking about separation from mother and from the parents in their coupling relationship. However, the dreams also express her fear of being in that relationship with the hallucinated uncle. Helen attempts to stop feeding the hallucinated uncle and thus risks losing him. He then becomes more threatening, dangerous and very similar to the voices instructing her to cut herself when she is turning towards relationships with her caregivers. The hallucination seems to represent a need to keep the uncle, representing father, alive as a figure literally until Helena has repaired him. If the verdict is, 'He is dead', Helena faces a cruel superego saying, 'You have killed him.'

The dreams further suggest that she has found some safety in relation to the staff in the inpatient unit and me, represented by the friend in the car. This possibility of a link with 'a friend, a woman in the car who can help her' is set against the terror of being alone. Always Helena feared having a separate existence. Alone, separate from either the hallucinated uncle or the maternal caregivers, Helena is beset with persecutory anxieties. The harsh cruel superego creates these anxieties by accusing her of oral greed and oral incorporation of the aunt and uncle, representing the internalized parental couple.

Of course, I still imagine that Helena may actually have had a seductive relationship with this older uncle upon whose lap she may have sat. I wonder if, in Helena's mind, his death was contributed to by her own confused oral and oedipal desires and her hatred of him for abusing her. Certainly in the dream, sitting on the uncle's lap initially seems to provide some pleasurable relief to Helena as she viewed the coupling of the parents. Later, however, in her dream, Helena was accused of killing the uncle.

Helena, like so many girls with eating difficulties, repeatedly stated or queried, 'I'm not fat and ugly, am I? I am spotty. I am ugly. I am too fat.' She also complained, 'My teeth are too big.' I sense that the damaged internal parents and the persecutory guilt about her ugly, destructive oral greed, her biting feelings represented by feeling of having big teeth, contribute to her preoccupation with being fat and ugly. The internal mother is also damaged by Helena's greedy attempts to get inside mother and possess and devour her completely. Then it seems that Helena is 'too fat' with greedy impulses and feels her female body is 'ugly' in intrusive identification with damaged inter nal mother and father, the internalized parental couple. The damaged internal mother is connected with an introjected external mother who is in external reality fragile, depressed and damaged. When in external reality Helen faces the fact that her external parents exist as a couple who will go out to enjoy themselves leaving her, she identifies with the tyrannical qualities of the hal-lucinations and uses their tyrannical qualities as a protection against her per-secutory fears of being left alone. This is confirmed by her threatening remark to her parents: 'If you go out, I will kill the baby sitter and myself.'

I should say something at this point about Helena's external circumstances. Two years previously, her father's much-loved older brother had died at the end of a six month convalescence with Helena's family. This uncle was idealized by Helena and never adequately mourned by the family. In fact, the family told me that they all still smelt the uncle's scent all over the house. The family believe in ghosts and the youngest of the three children in the family claims to have seen some.

Helena had always been a perfect child, never protesting, never uttering views contrary to those of her mother. She would not even choose a dress different from her mother's choice. Helena's reaction to the first separation from mother, necessitated by the birth of her sister, was to sit completely still, as if in a trance, for 24 hours. In her adolescence Helena, like several other girls with hallucinations and eating disorders, had persuaded her parents that she was too anxious to be left alone in her bedroom. As a result, for an extended period, the parents had placated Helena's persecutory fears by allowing Helena to share the parental bed. Perhaps this stimulated her oedipal wishes, promoting more greed as well as persecutory guilt for having interfered with the parental couple's union.

At school Helena had been an excellent student, popular with her friends. There had been some bullying of Helena just prior to the earache. The family's unbearable trauma of the uncle bleeding to death in their home was exacerbated inside Helena, for she had seemingly projected her own violence onto father's voice shouting at the uncle. It is unclear what 'the pain in Helena's ear' meant for her psychologically. One could speculate that father's shouting may have contributed to a somatization of the voice, which hurt her ears and gave her an earache. Certainly there was no robust external containment strong enough to bear Helena's physical and psychological pain. Helena experienced the paediatrician's advice and her parents' decision to send her back to school as a rejection and as well as a confirmation that her internal parents were deaf and cruel.

Three months after discharge, Helena started once-a-week therapy walking normally, with a hand extended to potentially reach her mother's arm if unsafe. She is now walking into different rooms in her house without her mother. Although she seems happier, at times she suddenly has a very sad face and starts crying. She cries at times in her sleep as well. Helena still says that she will not tell her mother or me the really horrible dreams she has. She is unclear about why she won't, but I sense that she is worried the dreams will become real as she describes them. In a recent session she talked about how the people in a television programme walked from the television screen into the sitting room. Clearly it is still difficult for Helena to differentiate internal reality from external reality. They tend to merge one into the other.

In the following session, three months after leaving hospital, Helena said there was one dream, of the 'non-terrible variety' that she had not yet described to me:

> There is a father who has three children. He cuts out the brain of the mother and puts it into a vase. The brain can't move. It seems to be like a

human being. Later the brain talks like a person. It gradually grows. It becomes a person. It has arms, shoulders, but it doesn't have any legs.

I was struck by how horrible this 'non-terrible' dream felt to me and realized then why Helena wanted to keep her dreams private. They had such cruelty inside them.

This dream, like some of her other dreams, seemed to be re-working the trauma that Helena had undergone. She seemed to be psychologically resident inside a mother whose brain was robbed by the father in a sadistic intercourse. I told Helena, 'You have had almost all your thinking capacity destroyed during her illness, losing memory, the capacity to read, write or do maths. You have also been imprisoned in some way, unable to eat, walk, have pleasure or live.' I also described,

> Perhaps you have felt very much like this mother in the dream. I think in this dream you are trying to work through the trauma of residing psychologically inside this mother captured and attacked by this father. In the dream you are describing what happened to you. You lost the capacities to live and work. Now you are recovering your will to live, recovering your capacities to think and dream about your emotional experiences. You are working with me to understand yourself.

Helena responded by saying, 'I feel ugly and fat.' She also stated, 'I want to stay home forever.' In a livelier tone, she added, 'But when I feel better I'd like some roller skates.' I talked about her contradictory wishes:

> On the one hand you want to stay locked inside the house, inside 'the mother', feeling ugly like this mother of the dream whom you got inside, possessed and controlled. Your other wish seems to be to move away from your own mother at home and from me, giving me and you, the mother and you, the freedom to separate from one another and live fully. The problem is that separating means suffering. Separating means letting go of me, the mother, giving her freedom to have pleasure with the father. It seems you want to be free, but don't quite yet know how to find the capacities to face this agony of separation. You need to feel stronger, more resilient inside first.

In Helena there has been a regression to a more primitive level of development as though in her developing through to her adolescence there had been a split in her personality with a part of herself developing ordinarily and a part still suffering a failed internalization of a good parental couple. The internal father seems to be a cruel figure, very intertwined with the maternal figure. In the earlier dreams Helena is accused of eating up and killing the father disguised as uncle, representing the breast, and the mother. In a dream Helena is also accused of greedily devouring the parental couple.

The hallucination protects Helena from the persecutory terror linked with depressive pain concerning her devouring attack on the father. Through the hallucination she keeps an exciting sadomasochistic attachment to a father who is not allowed to die, who is kept alive, until some kind person enables her to repair this internal father. Of course, at this primitive regressed level, there is a feeling that the father, represented by the uncle, needs to be concretely brought to life, but this is impossible. Only reparation of the internal father is possible (Rey, 1994).

In the dream there is a representation of Helena's introjection of the kind friend to whom she can turn for help. This 'kind friend', representing me and the keyworker nurse, enables Helena to begin to review the story of the damage of her internal figures. This is the internal damage which led to her incapacity to walk, talk, think, remember or find words for objects and people or recognize letters or numbers. In other words, attack on the internal mother, perceived as the father taking the mother's brain out, led to a damaged internal mother. Helena's baby self was in intrusive identification, imprisoned inside this attacked mother. Helena's actual mind became identified with this damaged brain.

The review of the story of damage to her internal figures commences when Helena develops a trusting relationship with her keyworker and me, her psychotherapist. She is able to begin to use dream-life not only to evacuate parts of her personality, but also to begin to think about her internal situation. Slowly Helena begins to integrate some of her disowned possessiveness and control. This is impeded to some extent by the presence of a fragile, damaged and immobile external mother to whom she repeatedly asks, 'Are you all right, mum?' She feels she hurts her mother by letting her mother know about the aggressive feelings existing within her and feels very worried about breaking her external mother down and prompting her mother to become too depressed and too unhappy. At times she has said to her mother, 'I comfort you, but why do you cry when I am distressed and come to you for help?' Here there is shown a mixture here of paranoid and depressive anxiety in relation to her mother's fragile state.

In her therapy, as I accept and interpret Helena's disappointment, disapproval, annoyance with me while I remain strong and understanding, Helena is gradually able to acknowledge some of her dislikes and hostile feelings toward me. Her dreams are still lurid and often a place into which she evacuates undigested violent and persecutory fears. At other times Helena slowly begins to be conscious of parts of her personality previously lodged in the dreams and hallucinations. She is becoming a more integrated and sane person. I still live with a sense that in order to overcome her jealousy of the parental couple, somehow she and the uncle became sexually involved, but that notion has never been verified.

During the ten months after leaving the inpatient unit, Helena came alone to her once-weekly psychotherapy. She has re-learned the alphabet and the names of objects as well as struggled to regain fine motor control to write and draw. She now reads with comprehension and solves maths problems with some difficulty. She has regained her normal weight, is walking and a few weeks ago she went out to practise riding on her bike. Each week she writes to her old friends who left the inpatient unit. However, Helena's mother was not yet willing to separate from Helena so she still had home tutoring. One year after leaving hospital Helena was attending a special day school on a full-time basis without her mother.

The hallucinatory experiences of the four other severely anorectic girls were similar to Helena's. The hallucinations were created at a point of separating from mother or therapist upon whom the girl depended. The hallucination was created when the inner child had a damaged, unsupportive and non-understanding internal mother and was thus needing to cling onto the external figure for security. For this reason, a primitive terror was experienced when facing separations. As time went on the hallucinations became more powerful and imbued with more parts of the Self.

In terms of interpretation, I found it essential to treat the hallucinatory figures with respect and thus acknowledge the child's sense of their emotional reality. Sometimes the girl was clearly aware that this experience which felt real, not like a 'hallucination', made others consider her to be 'crazy'. Therefore, this fear of 'being crazy' also needed to be understood. I attempted to get to know the hallucinatory figures without prejudice about their value. This enabled each girl to explore the nature of her relationship with the hallucinations. Gradually each girl was able to notice if there was a masochistic submission to the tyranny of the hallucinatory figure and she found a way out of her imprisonment by the hallucinations.

In the case of Amelia, aged 14, described by Segal and Magagna in the French article entitled 'Attachment to the false object' (1989), there is also a gradual transformation of the hallucinatory figure which Amelia experienced first at a moment of separation from the therapist. Initially Amelia experienced a hallucinated cruel figure with a knife, but later there appeared a more idealized beautiful queen. Subsequently, before the hallucinations were relinquished there was a more ordinary woman. Before inner containment of certain emotional experiences such as violent rage and before internalization of the therapist's helpful capacities, they seemed to be portrayed first in the hallucinated figures. Later there was more integration into a more established inner personality structure. Gradually Amelia began to find ways of living with the frustrations of life by remaining outside her hallucinatory world. This involved Amelia in discovering a capacity to love the primary figure more deeply, to allow the primary figure her freedom and to be resilient enough to experience the pain of separation from the helpful maternal figure.

The work brought into focus the need for careful monitoring of the therapist's countertransference in relation to Amelia's attachment to the tyrannical hallucinated figure. In particular, Amelia maintained an idealized relationship to the therapist and adhesively clung to and at times identified with the tyr-annical figure at the moment the therapist departed. The first phase of work required the therapist to describe the hallucinated tyrant as perceived by the patient, rather than locating the unbearable aggression within the patient. For example, Amelia was told by 'the tyrant' that she was not allowed to be happy, to eat, to read or to listen to music. She knew the tyrant, whom she called 'It', would be waiting for her at the end of her session with the thera-pist. The therapist explored with Amelia how the tyrant took her over the minute the therapist disappeared. The therapist described how Amelia clung to 'the tyrant' for a sense of safety.

The second phase of the work was to give Amelia some hope that through working with the therapist it would be possible to free herself from the tyr-ant's imprisonment. At this point it was important to show Amelia how she lost any notion of the therapist's internal capacities such as her concern and her thoughtfulness regarding her when they were separated. It was crucial for the therapist first to help Amelia hold onto their work and the prospect of their next meeting. Later the therapist gradually described how the therapist's different attributes were spoiled by the attacks of 'the little Amelia' both during and after the sessions. In the context of a loving, emotionally con-taining experience in thinking with her therapist, after some time Amelia was finally able to acknowledge her 'cruel self' and reply, 'At last, it took long enough for someone to see!'

Adolescence with its upsurge of bodily sensations and desires brings the anxiety about loss of control. The hallucinatory figure can be utilized as a kind of harsh superego figure maintaining control over the greedy, possessive desires. In another paper, 'Psychotherapy with an obsessional fourteen-year-old anorectic girl' Magagna (1987) I have described how Caterina progressed through a particular sequence of relationships with her 'three hallucinated witches' voices' before relinquishing them.

When I met 14-year-old anorectic Caterina, she was extremely emaciated. Unlike Helena, who was mute apart from her chanting on the unit, Caterina bombarded me with words until I felt myself to be a mother emptied by her child's wish to have everything immediately. Caterina confirmed my sensation with a dream of dying, entering heaven and being in a non-stop conversation with God. She was the only person allowed to be in heaven with God! She also dreamt of having a room to herself where she could eat non-stop without anyone looking. This representation of a wish to invade the maternal figure and have a non-stop feed was counteracted by Caterina's obsessional starva-tion diet which compelled her to eat only one bite of a morsel of food a minute for ten minutes.

The dictators of this obsessional diet were three hallucinatory voices, which were harsh superego-like witches. They controlled every minute of Caterina's life. For example, at 6:24 she was to awaken, at 6:26 she got out of bed, at 6:27 she put her clothes on and so on until 7:15 am when she could eat the first bite of toast and 7:16 when she could eat a second bite of toast. The witches dictated the terms of her life. Lacking any inner containment of her impulses, Caterina depended on these voices almost completely to keep her functioning somewhat normally. It was essential for me to enable Caterina to think in a serious, non-critical way about these voices which she experienced harsh voices of live dominating witches. I noted with her, 'It is interesting how you always seemed to listen to them. You completely submit to them.' I was able to understand when Caterina explained, 'The voices shout at me if I do not obey them completely.' In other words, working together, the sane part of Caterina and I found a way of initially describing the cruelty of the 'voices' and Caterina's sense that she had no option but to submit to them.

I felt myself at times very left out and insignificant in comparison to 'the voices'. I realized that it was important to note the moment in the sessions in which Caterina referred to the witches' voices. It seemed that they were often mentioned at the moment she might have the possibility of understanding something I said. They also occurred when she nodded as though she was depending on my understanding and feeling I might be important for her development. I wondered, 'Do you dare to confront these voices?' As time went on, I wondered with her, 'Maybe you might feel courageous enough to block your ears to the voices?' Gradually the sane Caterina seemed to gain more understanding of her desperate plight and she cried in the session saying she wanted to be 'normal' and live without the voices.

Caterina's psychological development could be assessed through looking at how she related to 'the voices' and how the quality of 'the voices' changed. As she began to appreciate the therapy, her appreciation of me seemed to be projected into the voices so that over time they became more benevolent. I silently associated them to Joan of Arc's helpful voices. I felt these changes were reflections of as yet unintegrated developing goodness and protective strength *nearly ready* to be internalized from good understanding experiences with me, her therapist. They also suggested the potentiality of diminishing harshness in her own superego.

Over time I could trace these five fairly distinct developments in the types of dialogue which Caterina had with the voices whose characteristics changed as she became psychologically healthier.

- As I am talking with her, Caterina hears the cruel voices dictating orders to her, threatening her with complete starvation if she disobeys them. They shout at her until she cries because of their loudness. She feels herself to be a helpless victim of their cruelty. They threaten her with death. They are so loud she wants to kill herself to get rid of them.
- While in my presence, Caterina says she feels imprisoned by the voices, but begins to feel slightly antagonistic towards them. She has the courage to tell me that she really doesn't like them much although she can't let them go. She cannot yet talk back to them.

- Caterina begins to disobey the voices and talks to her fellow students at school. She is beginning to have some hope that she can have a life with friends; however, when she disobeys the voices they threaten her and they put her on a concentration camp schedule of rising early, starving, following the old rigid routine of minute-by-minute procedures for living her life. This makes her feel despair.
- The voices seem to get somewhat kinder, less frequent, less intrusive, less pervasive. They seem to have less power to grab Caterina's attention, because her psychotherapy is becoming a base of security for her. The problem is that when she is disappointed with me she can easily turn to these destructive voices as allies against me.
- The voices disappear much of the time. They appear intermittently but only at times when Caterina is alone. At those moments when she is alone Caterina sometimes becomes panicked and feels lonely without the voices. At this later stage of therapy, before her own internal objects are more benevolent and functioning as a source of internal security, Caterina finds herself turning to a hallucinated substitute: the therapist's 'good voice' is being used keep her company. However, the voices often continue to tell Caterina not to eat, but now that she knew them better and could acknowledge their cruelty, she began to be active rather than passive in relation to them. She told them, 'You are boring. Leave me alone!' She also began to ignore their commands to stay alone. Instead she began to move from her isolated position and talked to students at school. She also began to swear at the voices.
- As Caterina began to own and integrate some of her own aggression, albeit to the 'voices', they changed in quality. They became more benevolent voices, at one moment, they even expressed surprise that food tasted good. Later they lost their influence over Caterina.

Caterina's experience demonstrates how terrifying it is for a young person to let go of the death wish represented by the destructive voices prompting suicidal despair. For example, if the young person's attachment is to this destructive part, as was the case with Caterina, the patient fears that losing *the destructive part* will result in *falling to pieces*.

In thinking about the hallucinations, I have begun to ask some questions facilitated by Henri Rey's (1994) work in *Universals of Psychoanalysis*. I wonder about what part of the Self, and what development level, is present in relation to what internal figure. Subsequently I have asked about the purpose and effect of part of the Self turning to the hallucination. I then question, what effect turning to the hallucinations has on the external object relations and what effect of the internal object relations have on the hallucinations. Here are some of the impacts of hallucinations which I have begun to understand:

- The baby part of the patient is intruding into the idealized father, mother or siblings. In other words, there may be a baby part hallucinating a good experience of a non-stop feed in heaven as in the case of Caterina.
- The baby part is in relation to the damaged maternal object, which is torn apart by separation from the baby, or damaged by infantile rage. For example, there may be a vision of a dead or bleeding mother as was the situation for Helena.
- The baby part is turning away from the dread of the persecuting damaged object to a perverse sexualized object. In this situation there may be the exciting, idealized big man who becomes a tyrant, like Helena's uncle.
- The entire Self can be a passive victim of harsh superego critic exerting obsessive control of both libidinal and destructive thoughts and actions, as shown by the witches' dictating and succeeding in controlling the girl's actions and eating every minute of her day. They threaten severe punishment if she disobeys. Caterina's hallucinations functioned in this way.
- The baby part is turning to an idealized object, which may be containing projected good aspects of a developing good internal object which cannot yet be integrated and internalized. This occurred when Amelia had a hallucination of a Madonna while splitting off infantile destructive wishes to the maternal figure.
- The 'ego ideal' empowers the Self to be generous, strives for some good, bears the pressure of eternal trauma, or simply is courageous. This is shown by Joan of Arc's voices, which prompted her to be sufficiently courageous to defend her country.

What impressed me as I reviewed the psychotherapy of the five adolescents with severe eating difficulties and hallucinations was how, in each situation, the adolescent daughter protected her somewhat fragile external mother, lacking a supportive husband, by not directly expressing hostility to her but rather expressing the hostility to the internalized mother. Meanwhile, the adolescent daughter suffered the enormous consequences of having a damaged external mother, an attacked internal mother and the need to hold onto and protect her relationship with her external mother. Also the girl felt ugly in intrusive identification with an attacked internal mother. Feeling terrorized or depressed without a good internal mother, she attached herself to hallucinatory figures that imprisoned her. With the presence of the hallucinations, the girl's living human links frequently remained starved of truth. At the same time the imprisoned anorectic's body suffered from malnutrition. The therapist's capacity to receive her primitive terrors, destructive feelings and projections of intense loving and hating feelings on a firm, thoughtful way enabled the anorectic girl to integrate split-off destructive aspects of herself previously present in her hallucinations.

Thus the anorectic girl was able to bear the frustration involved in holding an emotional experience and lending it thought through dreams and conversations with the therapist.

The hallucinations have included images of damaged internal objects as well as wish-fulfilling images. They have also been substitute companions during a solitary period in the form of internal objects, which were idealized figures, destructive tyrants and/or harsh superego critics. During each girl's therapy the hallucinations were modified and diminished considerably.

Conclusion

During the course of this chapter, I have begun an exploration of various types of hallucinatory figures and voices experienced by three adolescent girls with severe eating difficulties. These hallucinations are perhaps experienced only by a small minority of eating disordered girls who have an underlying psychotic or border-line-psychotic psychopathology. Nevertheless, it is important to consider them for they are often hidden and may facilitate understanding of some of the eating disordered young people's obedience to cruel thoughts prompting starvation.

Chapter 6

Suicidal and self-harm ideation accompanying eating disorders

In this chapter I shall describe predisposing and precipitating factors linked with self-harm and suicidality. I shall also discuss the self-harming person's differing relationships with internalized and external significant others. Consideration will also be given to some important clinical implications including understanding one's countertransference as well as the child's dreams and drawings for assessment and treatment of children and young people who are suicidal or who have self-harmed or attempted suicide.

Introduction

Elisa loves her husband who no longer loves her.

> Her baby is crying for her; turning away, Elisa walks slowly up the stairs. She is supposed to take the box filled with wooden clothes pegs, pull the pieces of washing out of the basket, one by one and hang them all along the line. And then? Another task to do. Why? With what aim in view? For no reason at all – there is no aim. And at the end of the day what will happen? Nothing. And tomorrow? The same as today. No, she just cannot do it.
>
> She has one thought. Just wait, don't give up on yourself, just wait! But Elisa doesn't think, doesn't hear, doesn't see. She feels only this strange void all around her. She cannot live without her love – even for a single day.
>
> She moves forward, her arms outstretched, groping along in a dead world in which she can no longer find her place. Elisa raises her hands, grips the window frame, climbs up onto the narrow sill: she is so tall that she has to bend her head a little so as not to touch the beams. For a moment she leans her cheek against the plaster of the wall, her eyes closed, her face serene, smiling almost. Eyes still shut, she will lean out a little, and in a slow, impassioned gesture, let go the hands that hold her in life.
>
> Elisa has lost not only the love of Gilles, her husband, but more importantly, her love for him. As her love for him is the only justification for her existence, she is in effect already dead, gazing into the abyss. When Elisa no longer is anything, she no longer wants to be anything anymore.[1]

DOI: 10.4324/9781003044970-7

This passage from Madeleine Bourdouxhe's (1992) novel, *La Femme De Gille*, illustrates the theme of this chapter, which is that attacks on the self, including annihilation, come when love dies. In every suicide, every attack on life, we must acknowledge the multi-faceted violence, the murdering of the body, of the psyche and of the designated internalized external object of the killing impulse.

As a child, adult and family psychotherapist in Great Ormond Street Hospital I have witnessed the following:

- An 18-month-old child consistently turning his head away from mother as she attempts to give him a spoon of food, necessary for life.
- A 15-year-old girl rarely opening her eyes and not eating, speaking or moving.
- Four anorectic young people from 12 to 18 years, all of whom have said 'I just want to die' not only in words but also in their not eating, over-dosing, and self-harming actions.

Throughout all these current experiences I have been trying to understand these young people who are expressing the wish to die, slowly dying by not eating, and sometimes actively attempting to cut or kill themselves. Research shows that at the time of referral almost half of the young people suffering from anorexia nervosa are clinically depressed.

In this chapter I shall describe aspects of therapeutic work with these young people who, unable to have or to maintain a loving attachment to a good internal object, attach themselves to destructive forces within. I will begin by showing the enormous variation in the intensity and quality of the young people's destructive impulses, the nature of their relationship to the internal object, and the conscious and unconscious intentions underlying their self-harm and/or attempted suicide. Subsequently, I will indicate precipitating and predisposing factors, including certain types of dreams, which suggest a lack of a good internal object and/or an addiction to the destructive part of the self. Such factors should prompt a clinician to be particularly concerned about the risk of suicide or the reoccurrence of a suicide attempt. Lastly, I shall describe important treatment issues which individual psychotherapists and multidisciplinary teams should consider when working with depressed young people.

Throughout the chapter I shall intersperse vignettes of therapeutic work with these self-harming, suicidal, non-eating children and young people.

Transference and countertransference issues

From a psychological point of view, attacks on life are very complex. In order to understand self-harming, suicidal young people, I must understand not only their feelings about themselves and their parents, but also their feelings about the professional staff involved in their treatment. I realize that at the time of any young person's threatened attack on life, I also need to understand the parents' and my and other hospital professionals' current feelings towards the young person. In addition, I must understand both our attitudes subsequent to an attack on life and our attitudes that fluctuate as the young person's self-destructive ideation and activity persists (Campbell and Hale, 2017).

Questions to ask regarding the transference–countertransference relationship

Dr Henri Rey (1994), former Maudsley Hospital Consultant Psychiatrist and Psychoanalyst, suggests that these questions are important to ask at the time of any self-harm or thoughts of self-harm:

- What part of the young person is involved?
- In what emotional state?
- Situated where in space and time?
- Does what?
- With what motivation?
- To what part of the significant other?
- In what state?
- Situated where in space and time?
- With what consequences for the significant other?
- And with what consequences for the young person?

I will use Dr Rey's questions to help analyse the relationship of the patient to the therapist in the following psychotherapy session:

Susan's session

Eighteen-year-old Susan said she wanted to torture me. She felt I simply couldn't understand how hurt she was. Arriving early for her session, Susan had seen my previous patient leave the session and get into the car with her mother. Being raised in an emotionally and sexually abusing, neglectful and poor income family, Susan had had to depend on herself. Seeing my previous patient get into a comfortable car with her mother stirred up all Susan's feelings of isolation, loneliness and envy. After she seated herself in the session, Susan complained fiercely, 'You simply do not realize how lonely I am, how alone I have felt during all my life. You won't ever be able to comprehend that!' Susan felt certain that she could tell that my middle-class background was different from hers and she indicated that I probably had had caring parents. Then she was silent.

I replied, 'You feel I am all that you have. It feels so unfair, so painful, when you see the girl with her mother. It makes you furious. I am trying to help you have more in your life … You have found therapy and that is helping you to have a better life.'

At the end of the session Susan remained seated, refusing to leave the room. I said, 'You need to look after the little girl that wants to stay always with me and now has to leave. I understand that is very difficult.' Still Susan didn't move from her chair. Becoming worried, I then added, 'You seem to be not allowing space for the next person who will come to see me. She is to feel as pushed out as you feel.' Susan still remained immobile, so I also wondered, 'Would you rather have the next person see you with me for then you could spoil her session the way you feel yours has been spoilt?' Susan got up and, very uncharacteristically, she threw her chair hard against the door, which was still shut. This created a startling bang, which was accompanied by the seat of the chair falling off. I was visibly startled.

Then Susan rushed out of the room, shouting, 'I hate you and I am going to kill myself!' Susan had deliberately left her diary on the floor, giving me the anxiety-provoking message that it wouldn't be needed anymore.

Subsequently, one and a half hours later, Susan phoned me. She apologized, saying, 'I am sorry for being so out of control.' After a pause, she shared, 'I am all right. I am calling from a railway station.' I asked, 'What is the matter? What is happening?' Susan said that she couldn't talk as she had to rush to get the train.

I wasn't at all clear where she was going, for she lived near the consulting room; however, she had gone to visit a friend and safely returned for the next session. Later, as I pondered over Susan's suicide threat, I asked:

What part of her is speaking? An infant.

In what emotional state? Feeling jealous of the girl who has a protective mother caring for time, feeling abandoned at the end of sessions, feeling helpless in the face of this painful hurt, envy and overwhelming rage.

Situated where in space and time? She arrives to feel my lap soiled by others and departs feeling I am insensitive, like a hard, shut door and she is left to go into a cold outside place.

Does what? Attacks, injures 'my lap', my heart, the chair and my door, representing the boundaries to the session, particularly the ending of the session.

With what motivation? To attack my uncaring heart and non-understanding mind so I can feel and understand her pain. She also wishes 'to bang her feelings into thick-skinned me', penetrating me so that I feel deeply hurt.

To what part of the object? My lap, my heart, my mind, my boundaries.

In what state is the object? My lap is soiled, my heart is felt to be hard, my mind is experienced as non-comprehending.

With what consequences to the significant other? My heart is shocked and hurt and I feel extremely worried about Susan. I am aware in her phone call she leaves me 'shut out'.

And with what consequences to the young person? Susan initially feels pleasure and relief from the feelings which have overwhelmed her thoughtful self.

Subsequently she becomes extremely worried that, because of her attack, I will abandon her and that she will lose a loving contact with a 'good me' inside herself. Her phone call suggests Susan also feels sorry that she has been very worrying and hurtful to me.

It is crucial to ask these questions when a young person makes a threat to kill herself. Such a threat represents an attack on the internalized and external therapist once felt to be good and now felt to be hard and uncomprehending, an attack on the significant others in the young person's life, as well as a possible physical attack on her own life.

Six of the observable phenomena in attacks on life

In answering the questions Rey posed regarding the suicidal young person's relationships, I have noted six rather distinct relationship patterns:

- The young person in an active, deliberate way *chooses death*.
- The young person *uses the threat* of suicide.
- The young person through suicidal thoughts *retreats from* feeling persecuted in her life.
- The young person *is threatened by destructive voices* demanding and threatening the self with death, but she still feels slightly separate rather than completely identified with these voices or thoughts.
- The young person is *overwhelmed by feelings and by destructive voices* and passively submits to the death impulse. Often there is some sense that the body may be destroyed, but the soul might be entering a better place than in her life. In other words, a denial of actual death is present.
- The young person *tries to recover the self* through hurting or killing the body. She is so depersonalized at this point that the self-destructive phantasies are not fully acknowledged as hurting the self; rather, they represent an attempt integrate the disintegrated personality and locate the sane mind.

Further exploration of the six types of relationships underlying suicide or self-harm

The young person in an active, deliberate way chooses death

John Bowlby (1969) states that a child's suicide attempt is a response to the loss of a good relationship to an external attachment figure. The suicide attempt may also represent a lack of a secure attachment to a good internal figure, a situation based either on the lack of opportunity to have sufficiently good experiences with a satisfactory attachment figure or loss of the good internalized parents due to the incapacity to bear frustration and subsequent destructive attacks on the primary attachment figures who are subsequently internalized. Any one of these experiences may prompt the majority of the adolescents attempting suicide to feel there is nothing good left in them, and no one good left their lives. No love is left. They perceive the external environment to be unresponsive and/or abusive in some way. Furthermore, prior to the suicide or self-harm they do not experience sufficiently good enough internal parents. This lack of a good *internal object* makes it impossible for them to sustain the perceived lack of love and sense of rejection by the *external attachment figures* represented, in the transference, by the therapist.

I have given examples of this experience of 'nothing being left', no love left, in the story of Elisa, described in the beginning of the chapter. As in the suicide of Elisa, young people, such as those in the films *Adele H.* and *The Lacemaker*, might kill themselves when abandoned by their lovers. Lacking the security of previously established good internal objects, they depend almost completely on their lovers. When abandoned, such girls, now left without any good internal objects, are filled with only a sense of hate which creates even more of a sense of bad abandoning objects. Thus they experience 'nothing being left' and they can become suicidally depressed. Their experience can be expressed by these words:

The beauty of love has not found me.
Its hands have not gripped me so tight.
For the darkness of hate is upon me.

Hate, rather than love and sadness for what is lost, creates a sense of profound despair of 'having nothing'.

In the hospital, Amelia, aged 15, is suffering from anorexia nervosa, masking a psychotic depression. She is described in more detail in Chapter 5. During the Easter holidays, Amelia takes an overdose of tablets, saying that all she wants is to die. She actively chooses to kill herself.

What part of her choses this death? Amelia's uncaring adult part.

In what emotional state? The infantile self suffers a sense of abandonment by her key worker, the nurse, her therapist.

Does what? Threatens abandoning figures felt to be cruel in leaving her.

With what motivation? To attack the cruel figures leaving her.

With what consequences for the inner object? The inner object is further attacked and becomes a cruel uncaring figure.

With what consequences for herself? Amelia attacks her Self physically and emotionally.

With what consequences for external rescuing others? Amelia forces the 'designated rescuing others', the multidisciplinary inpatient team, to acknowledge the effects of their joint abandonment during the holiday. In the future, they will be more careful in planning spaced out holidays and working through the young people's feelings about their absences.

The young person uses the threat of death to save the self and avoid breakdown of defensive omnipotent thinking

When parents in an enmeshed relationship with their anorectic daughter attempt to provide firm boundaries and rules for the child, the parents sometimes seem to move from being helplessly impotent to unleashing their inhibited aggression and becoming harsh and physically punitive. Nine-year-old anorectic Alice does not obey her parents' exhortations to eat and to stay at home. When Alice throws a tantrum instead of obeying, her parents lock her in her room. Alice has built up a 'hard shell' of angry defiance, through which she attempts to protect her vulnerable self.

On these occasions when her parents become hard and punitive in their countertransference to their difficult anorectic child, Alice makes half-gestures towards suicide: she puts a plastic bag on her head, puts a rope round her neck, cuts her wrist with a knife. On one occasion when she is feeling very persecuted by me and her mother in a psychotherapy session, Alice makes a mock attempt to strangle herself with the tied up arms of her jumper. She asks her mother to pull the jumper arms to make the noose even stronger. In these activities, I felt Alice expresses at least three violent experiences: Firstly, Alice becomes 'like ice' to herself. She feels her parents, her family, and individual psychotherapists are hard, non-understanding figures, cold and insulated from tender feelings. Feeling a lack of love, Alice turns to a cold, unfeeling 'ice in her heart'. She becomes violent to herself; however, she succeeds in projecting her distress into us through an attacking, shocking event to pierce what she perceives as our hard, uncaring armour. Secondly, Alice attempts to split off her 'crazy' state of mind, and project it into me. In one session, she makes a drawing of a very distorted, persecuted face filled with voices dictating messages.

Meanwhile, she speaks in an intellectualized way, trying to remain aloof from her emotional experience. When Alice doesn't get her own way, she icily says, 'I get so upset I just feel I'll have an epileptic fit, go mad, or suicide.' It seems I am to contain the horror and terror of this crazy state, which Alice, through her emotional aloofness when drawing, attempts to split off and project into me. Thirdly, through her suicidal gestures and suicidal threats, Alice shows that she feels her omnipotent self, which she depends on for emotional safety, is being attacked and killed by external authoritarian controls. When there is an attack on this omnipotent self upon which she depends for security in lieu of the parents, the *omnipotent self* rears its cruel head, dictating to her, 'You don't need life, death is the answer. Everything will be nice then.'

In all three of these violent experiences, I, as the therapist, experience Alice's terror of death – death of her sane self, death of her *omnipotent self* protecting her, and death linked with her primitive infantile anxieties of dying. These infantile terrors of dying have never been sufficiently contained in Alice.

Since infancy, her terror of catastrophic death is dealt with through *omnipotent phantasies* instead of being dealt with through depending on the parental capacities for mentalization (Allen and Fonagy, 2006) and containment of her primitive anxieties.

I am suggesting that treatment interventions, including psychotherapy, inpatient treatment and feeding, which do not sufficient contain the child's anxiety about losing the *omnipotent protective armour* to hold the self together, might lead to destructive acting out. Rosenfeld (1987a) has described various functions of the omnipotent self to which the infant may cling to in moments of psychological adversity. Originally the *omnipotent self* might have offered the infant protection in relation to abusive relationships and pathological attachment relationships including emotionally uncontaining relationships. However, when overused, the *omnipotent self* becomes a *destructive omnipotent self*, which binds the healthy personality to it. By binding the healthy personality to it, the *omnipotent self* thus attacks the strength, goodness and vitality present in the relationship with the therapist. It doesn't allow access to the understanding of the therapist. It also attacks the young person's thoughtful self, trying to get in touch with intense feelings (Bion, 1962). Ultimately, the omnipotent self attacks the link with life through self-harm and/or suicide.

The young person retreats from persecutory figures

In a film of food-refusing children made by Professor David Skuse, one 18-month-old child is rejecting the gaze and refusing the food given by her mother. In his film, each food-refusing child has felt abandoned or misunderstood by the mother. Food refusal also implies that the child has never achieved a harmonious attunement (Stern, 1985) while trying to find love, nurturing, pleasure with an emotionally containing mother. Mother's mentalizing is required for healthy development of the baby. Mother's ability to mentalize for herself and the baby allows the baby to develop his/her own innate capacity for mentalization. By *mentalizing* I am referring to a process by which the person concerned holds emotions alive internally and through thinking gives meaning to the desires, needs, feelings, beliefs and reasons underlying interpersonal interactions.

A baby needs mentalizing more than simple basic comforts to stay psychologically healthy. Mother is perceived to be bad if she is depriving baby of a satisfactory, properly attuned emotionally containing relationship (Bion, 1962). As a result, anger to mother is projected unto her and her spoon. Mother and spoon are filled with baby's projections of aggression, resulting in baby's experience of spoon and mother being perceived as bad and persecutory. Subsequently the baby refuses mother's rhythm of caregiving and also refuses to open her mouth for mother's food. I am not saying that the mother is bad, but rather suggesting that the mother and baby are not in a harmonious relationship. Alongside a mis-attuned relationship with the mother, the child simultaneously begins to develop a style of using *omnipotent control*, a kind of pseudo-autonomy (Bick, 1968) in relationships. Omnipotent control is used in lieu of mentalization of feelings. Gradually the use of omnipotent control captures parts of the healthy self. Subsequently it becomes destructive and the base of obsessional control so prevalent in eating disordered young people.

The young person is threatened by destructive voices demanding and threatening the self with death, but she still feels slightly separate, rather than completely identified with these voices

Some young people have a destructive omnipotent self in the form of hallucinatory voices attacking healthy, intimate attachments to important figures in a young person's life. Caterina, a 14-year-old anorectic girl, already described in Chapter 5, begins telling me about the voices that haunt her. There are three voices; they are women's voices. They feel like the three cruel witch figures in *Macbeth*. They tell her what to do and threaten her if she doesn't obey or does the wrong thing. For example, at times the witchlike voices forbid her to eat anything. They criticize her if she does not follow her minute-by-minute programme for the day. When she leaves the therapy room, they criticize her for speaking to me. They are very forceful, cruel and demanding voices. She feels suicidal because she can't bear the loudness of the voices. Although her situation is extremely severe, a young person who is depressed, self-harming and/or suicidal may have less assertive destructive thoughts to which she turns when in a crisis or disappointed and hurt in the process of trying to establish a meaningful, helpful relationship with someone important to her. The therapist's work is to help the young person find a way of becoming cognisant of the moments when these destructive, omnipotent thoughts occur or become more potent. This is the first step in taking responsibility for them. The therapy to help Caterina fend off the luring appeals of the voices are described in Chapter 5.

The young person is overwhelmed by feelings accompanied by destructive voices, which demand submission to the death wish

Yufang suffered a depressive stupor. As she was Chinese and her parents spoke very poor English, we were not even certain whether or not she spoke English. Clearly it was not apparent from the times her eyes were open that she responded to the meaning of English words. To the observer, Yufang felt almost dead. It is difficult to know what happens to a dying girl who barely opens her eyes, let alone speaks. It seems to me that even the wish to die has wilted and become, instead of *a wish*, an overwhelming drowning in death or sleep. Although the psychotherapy sessions I offered to her were briefly successful and she began 'to awaken' and look at me, Yufang subsequently retreated into her former comatose state. I didn't know from her history how anorectic she might be, but now she was in a depressive stupor or pervasively retreating (Lask et al., 1991).

This 17-year-old Chinese girl had felt abruptly torn away from all that she knew: her culture, her friends, her boyfriend, her parents and her grandmother. She had nothing to which she could anchor herself in this new world in London. She had developed through holding onto external relationships without ever really internalizing the capacity to think about the feelings which she had. Her lifelong habit appeared to be using massive denial to cope with intense feelings of any kind.

Later, as she was recovering, Yufang told me about some former thoughts: The air was spinning round the earth. All the houses had fallen over. She said she felt like breaking through a glass window, throwing herself out of the window. At this moment, when she was so ill, I felt she was being submerged by the death impulse, enclosed in a dead object. Yet part of her had been trying to come to life with me. From the start of her depression, even though Yufang didn't speak, she required my thoughtful presence to move psychologically and physically towards life. Yufang's development is more fully described in Chapter 7.

With Sean, a psychotically depressed boy, the situation was slightly different. He slept. He was very drowsy, both because of drugs and because he retreated defensively into sleep. I again used the family dolls. Holding the dolls in my hands, I asked Sean if he could wake the Sean doll up. To my surprise, Sean awakened and took the 'mother doll' and pushed her towards the Sean doll and very cruelly awakened him.

I described, 'The Sean doll feels there is a cruel mother doll making the child do just what she wants.' I added, 'This mother doll doesn't care one jot about what her boy wants. The boy doll just wants to sleep and sleep and forget about everything.' Once he felt understood, Sean awakened fully with a smile.

In psychotic depression the *self is submerged by the death wish*. If I could, I would begin treating a psychotically depressed young person the day she was hospitalized. We prolong the illness by depriving the young person of the understanding she needs to hold onto or rediscover the wish to live. If we keep demanding speech from a young person, we drive her into a state of persecution. *First we must lend our understanding!*

In order to come to life, to emerge from being smothered by death, both these young people, Yufang and Sean, required a mentalizing adult, an adult who could bring emotional nourishment to their wilting and wasting Selves. It seemed essential that someone attempt to provide understanding of their wish to die, or their feeling submerged by the massive denial of sleep or the forceful death instinct. They could not live without an emotional rope gently tugging them to emotional life. After the first time she heard the story of her life, which I told using the doll family, Yufang was willing to be fed. She would not feed herself initially, but she would swallow food put into her mouth.

The young person tries to recover the self through hurting or killing the body

There are remarkable similarities between the psychic state during trauma and the mental state of some suicidal patients (Shneidman et al., 1976). Indeed, some suicide attempts and repeated self-mutilations may represent a means of interrupting the traumatic state (Simpson, 1976) and trying to find the sane self.

Both holocaust victims and suicidal patients describe a 'break in the life-line' and a 'loss of personality' (Venzlaff, 1964). When psychic numbing sets in, the person becomes aware of a feeling of 'deadness' and depersonalization. The internalized external figures are felt to be numb and uncaring to the self and the self is in identification with these hard, uncaring internalized figures. The self is then left psychologically surrendering to destructive craziness and a sense of psychological emptiness. It is this sense of being left with destroyed internal objects and a resulting state of emptiness which feels so lethal.

In this situation one often senses an overwhelming danger of loss of self. There is a blocking of, and dissociation from, one's experience. Self-observation, cognition and symbolic thought are reduced to a minimum. There is a sudden wish to make *a violent exit* from this state of helplessness and depersonalization through actively taking her own life. Or there may be a wish *to obtain relief* from this depersonalized state through cutting the self, or injuring the self in some other way. It is as though destroying the self or hurting the self provide solutions to the tension of being depersonalized. The razor can represent comfort and reassurance, a perverted form of self-care. However, repeated cutting ultimately only compounds and deepens the link with the *tyrannical destructive omnipotent self* enslaving the young person (Gardener, 2001).

Cutting may also help the young person feel 'real': Amelia, 15, said, 'I had to cut myself – I didn't know who I was before. I had to see the blood.' She needed to have a sense of a live object that could experience pain and a live self (Chapter 5). In her book, *Nobody, Nowhere*, Donna Williams (1992) wrote of experiences and feelings similar to Amelia's:

> At home I would spend hours in front of the mirror staring at my own eyes, whispering my name over and over, sometimes trying to call myself back. At other times I became frightened at losing my ability to feel myself. I was losing my ability to feel. My own world may have been a void, but losing my grip on it left me unmercifully in some sort of limbo without any feeling or comfort whatever. I began to hurt myself to feel something.

Depersonalization followed by self-harm or suicidal attempts can become addictive processes to a *tyrannical omnipotent self* which substitutes itself for being able to contain conflictual, painful, terrifying emotional experiences in relation to important caregivers.

The suicidal young person's motives in relation to potential rescuers

Alongside the wish to die is generally an unfulfilled wish to be rescued

The young person, through a suicide attempt, tries to restore the mother who has abandoned her. Who is the designated rescuer? Obviously it is the person (or people) to whom the young person is most attached. The *designated rescuer* is also the one upon whom the young person may originally have projected a great deal of aggression. The therapist – who is, in the transference, a representative of the original object – can be the specific *designated rescuer* as old or new traumas are experienced.

The designated rescuer is also the person whom the suiciding person unconsciously holds responsible for his own impending death

For example, imagine a young person who takes an overdose and then shouts at her mother, the object of her hostility, because she experiences her mother as being uncaring. Paradoxically, the young person still hopes that the mother will change from being the person she perceives as an uncaring mother and rescue her. Through the mother rescuing her, the young person hopes that she will experience herself as being actually loved and lovable. Also, through rescuing the child, showing compassion rather than hostility to her child, the mother shows that she actually cares about the child; she is not the 'bad' mother the girl tried to 'kill off'.

The request to the rescuer includes the need for the designated rescuer to be receptive to the threat of suicide

As Rey (1994) stated, it is important to assess the motivation of a suiciding person in relation to the *designated rescuer*. Although the young person attempting suicide has a perception of uncaring internalized external figures, usually the young person hopes that the *external designated rescuers* will transform themselves and be able to reach out to the victim, be empathic to the victim and be strong enough to recognize and acknowledge destructive impulses both in the suicidal young person *and* in the designated rescuer.

A dangerous designated rescuer

A *dangerous designated rescuer* is a person who implies consent or unconsciously colludes with the suicide. An actual attack on the body during the pre-suicidal state can be precipitated by an actual experience of rejection or a feeling of having been misunderstood, dismissed, or abandoned. The suiciding patient experiences rejection in a particularly potent way when the rejection is experienced in relation to someone who is valued. When the rescuer refuses to respond as unconsciously or consciously desired by the pre-suicidal person in need, the suicide occurs.

Those people working with depressed and suicidal individuals are vulnerable to being provoked or subtly led into attitudes and reactions that are experienced by the individual as rejection or collusion with the suicidal phantasy. In other words, prior to the suicide, the pre-suicidal person could have externalized the bad, uncaring, punitive internalized object relationship, thus prompting uncaring in the countertransference relationship with the *designated rescuers*. Of course in some situations the *designated rescuers* may simply be uncaring. Beware of professional defences against feeling deeply – this may lead to becoming perceived as a *dangerous rescuer*. On the other hand, feelings need to be tempered by thought and self-scrutiny, so therapists don't 'act out' in the countertransference.

Precipitating factors leading to self-harm or suicidal activity

External events *in the present* may act as precipitating factors which activate unconscious problems deriving from early relationship conflicts which have been internalized.

Real or perceived loss of concern of the caregivers

Real or perceived loss of care is a common factor precipitating suicide according to research findings published in 'Suicidal acts' (Campbell and Hale, 1991). A danger signal is the loss of concern which can be shown both by the suicidal person towards others, and by the others towards the suicidal person. One of the consequences of the suicidal individual's withdrawal from other people during a pre-suicidal phase, albeit behind a deceptive façade of sociability, is that the depressive affects, anxieties and fears are no longer communicated. As a result, those around the suicidal person may cease to respond to her needs and feelings as they ordinarily might do. Even if they have some intellectual awareness of the suicidal risk at this critical moment, the young person's withdrawal cuts others off from responding to any normal stimulus for empathic responses of alarm or concern (Tähkä, 1978).

A suicide attempt may now be imminent because the young person is emotionally cut off from the friends, relatives or professional helpers who would ordinarily protect him from himself. Thus, he *both feels and is* more abandoned. The signal for this danger is the sudden loss of *subjective* emotional concern for a depressed or suicidal young person by those most involved with him. For the professional, the loss of concern may manifest itself as a failure to recognize the importance of the therapeutic relationship in the young person's life. For example, the therapist may react to the young person's narcissistic withdrawal by letting the young person temporarily stop his therapy or leave the inpatient unit. The young person then perceives the therapist as sanctioning and colluding with his suicidal phantasies. The therapist's reaction, of altering the therapeutic frame for work, then becomes an essential ingredient in the fulfilment of the suicide plan. Thus, the therapist should carefully scrutinize any impulse to alter his interpretive stance or collude with disruption of the consistency of the therapeutic setting – unless, of course, hospitalization is required. Whenever possible, the therapist should maintain the cardinal rule of maintaining the centrality and reliability of the therapeutic frame. This means having sessions for a particular length of time, at an exact regular time, on a particular day, with sufficient notice regarding any changes in the therapy schedule.

Another danger signal is the appearance of the therapist's countertransference reactions, which might be inappropriately influenced by the therapist being overwhelmed by his/her own traumatic life experiences. Such a countertransference may contribute to loss of empathy or failure to perceive a psychic homicide. A greater understanding of the danger signals of loss of emotional connectedness with the patient may enable the therapist to play a more constructive role during a pre-suicide state. Racker (1968) in his book *Transference and Countertransference* is very helpful in examining subtle aspects of pathological countertransference experiences. The danger is that if the signals are missed, the therapist, by being perceived as rejecting or non-understanding, may behave unwittingly as the hostile internal object from the past that the young person can only relate to through death.

Repetitious suicidal gestures on the part of the young person can often mean that the therapeutic team has not worked through some of the 'stuckness' in the therapist, in the treatment team and/or in the family system. For this reason, it is essential to be curious about the emotions underlying the interaction between the therapeutic team and the young person as well as between the young person and her parents and the parents and the therapeutic team. Using the questions of Rey (1994) outlined earlier in the chapter can be helpful in this process. It is difficult, but important for the therapeutic team members to have support in being honest about their own aloofness or aggression in relation to the young person or the young person's parents. Also a conflictual parental marriage prompts pathological interactions and defences in family members. Similarly, the therapeutic interaction between the young person and therapist can be detrimentally influenced by conflictual team dynamics. When anyone in the system surrounding the child is felt not to be properly attuned to and available to the young person, the young person can feel neglected and at risk of self-harm or suicide.

I have begun thinking of staff's relational difficulties which perpetuate oscillation between life and death in these young people who attack life. Here are some of my thoughts:

- If the staff says 'we want you to live' and strongly endeavour to make the young person hold onto the wish to live, the young person may project the wish to live solely into the staff and tug like mad in opposition, pulling towards death, suicide, killing wishes.
- If the staff have difficulty bearing the patient's hatred and aggression because they don't feel good about themselves, they may respond to attacks on their caring by being hurt, rather than by recognizing the young person's cruelty towards them. The patient may then feel that her cruelty is uncontained and uncontainable and cannot be shown to the therapist or other staff members. The young person may then retreat to cruel treatment of herself.
- If the staff allow themselves to be cruelly or contemptuously treated by the young person and then harden themselves in order not to feel hurt by the young person, the young person may feel that she is not able to make a deep enough impact on staff. She may then feel that she has to cut through the 'tough skin' of the staff by cutting her body in a way that has a permanent effect on everyone.
- Getting better means standing alone and facing one's destructiveness towards oneself, the staff, the family. Letting go of the death wish means facing depressive pain about one's own cruelty. Both the therapist and the young person will need to relinquish the defences erected against experiencing the psychic pain of recognizing cruelty in the self and the other.
- It is impossible for the young person to 'let go of the addiction to the death wish' until there is a possibility and a capacity to depend upon a caregiver who is experienced as reliable, trustworthy, empathic and attuned caregiver. Losing the symptoms of self-harm and/or suicidal ideation involves *a terrifying 'letting go'* of a method of *controlling significant others' involvement* and depending on *significant others* as reliable, emotionally containing and therapeutic caregivers.

For the young person, 'getting better' does involve *losing the significant caregivers* in the inpatient unit and eventually ending outpatient psychotherapy. Thus 'getting better' requires time to find a separate space outside the secure prison of the addiction to the destructive omnipotent self, time to find a separate space outside the inpatient unit and also time to find a separate Self who can exist without psychotherapy. In Great Britain, a survey of 850 people showed that those people who weren't followed up appropriately (after seven days or not at all) after leaving psychiatric hospital were twice as likely to attempt suicide and a third more likely to harm themselves compared to respondents who said they were followed up within seven days of being discharged (Mind, 2017). This means it is essential to pay particular attention to the need for the time and the therapeutic opportunity to internalize the mentalizing capacities of the therapeutic team and mourn their loss. Likewise, it is important to make sufficient preparation for separations of any kind, by giving exact dates of therapists' and caregivers' absences or departures, patients' date for leaving hospital or ending psychotherapy.

In summary, young people can appear more psychologically healthy in the containing atmosphere of the inpatient unit than they actually will be in the community. The loss of the *containing presence, the mentalizing significant other*, is a *significant loss* for a young person.

Loss of significant attachment figures

Adolescence is a particularly turbulent time. Laufer (1995) describes the factors precipitating suicide in adolescence. He highlights the fact that the young person's adolescent developmental task of establishing relationships outside the home and becoming more independent of the external parents requires the young person to depend on sufficiently good internalized parents with the capacity to face psychic pain and mentalize about important feelings.

Apart from this experience of gaining increased independence of parents, a young person who has lost an attachment figure is more prone than others to consider suicide. Bowlby (1969) states that the motives for attempting or completing a suicide can best be understood as responses to the actual loss or threatened loss of an attachment figure.

Mobilization of aggression to the body and the mind

As described in the outline of Rey's (1994) points for consideration, the suicidal young person mobilizes her aggression to her own body but the motivation for doing so is linked with relationships to both *external significant others* and *internalized significant others*. The personal motivation for the aggression involves a wish for some kind of rescue from the *psychic pain of loss*. The process of losing a significant other involves experiencing a sense of abandonment by *a significant other*. This is often accompanied by a reaction of hatred and anger about the loss of the *significant other*. The hatred and anger towards *the significant other* results in internalization of an attacked and thus damaged *significant other*. A persecutory, punitive guilt related to the destructive impulses may then ensue. For example, an internal Hitler figure, created by aggressive impulses towards *significant others*, may demand death. Or, in order to protect the *external significant other* from bodily damage, the young person may attack the *body self* identified with *internalized significant others*. Another motivating factor is the creation of a sense of non-existence prompted by the destruction of loving links with both internalized and external *significant others*.

Experiencing a psychotic depression

A psychotic depression occurs when the young person fully identifies with the attacked and damaged lost object. The process leading to psychotic depression in a young person involves a repeated re-enactment of hostility to the *significant others*, usually the parents (or the therapist representing them in the transference), accompanied by a subsequent identification with the attached and damaged internalized objects. The Self is subsequently treated as though it were the hated, frustrating object. Hostility towards the frustrating external object is repeatedly turned into hostility directed to the Self identified with the internalized object. Both the wish to murder the internalized object and the persecutory guilt about one's aggression can eventuate in suicide. The risk of suicide is *often greater* as the young person is in the recovery process, less depressed and being more conscious of the hostility underlying the psychotic depression.

Predisposing factors

It is important to differentiate precipitating factors for self-harm and suicide from predisposing factors. Laufer (1995) describes three basic predisposing factors:

- Feeling sexually abnormal in some way.
- Fearing engulfment in a relationship with a family member that threatens one's sense of identity. For example, the child in a symbiotic relationship who experiences this family member as existing more independently may equate this with separation or desertion. The parents' divorce or an unexpected death of this family member may also have this same impact. Subsequently the child finds ways of trying to get rid of unbearable pain in various ways including self-harming or killing oneself.
- Fearing abandonment which prompts feelings of self-hatred and self-denigration.

In all three situations, the person experiences the lack of a secure sense of Self, identified with an internal containing good object. This means that the capacity for tolerating and thinking about painful emotional experiences is limited and feelings tend to overwhelm the sense of Self. In addition to Laufer's general research findings, there are other specific factors predisposing a young person to kill herself, which include the following.

Sexual abuse

Suzanne Sgroi's (1982) research into sexual abuse revealed that in one ongoing group of sexually abused girls, *every* adolescent who had been subjected to an incestuous relationship experienced suicidal feelings. The suicidal ideation ranged from taking a few aspirins and just becoming sick, to one member who threw herself naked into an ice-filled river. The girls in the study reported that they had felt suicidal feelings to be a taboo subject to discuss because they had created enough problems already by disclosing the incest. Following disclosure, each girl felt intense suicidal feelings for six reasons:

- She felt responsible and guilty for her incestuous sexual behaviour.
- She felt responsible for the disclosure and its impact on others.
- She felt responsible for the disruption of the family.
- She felt shame about the incest itself and about disclosing it.
- She felt her body, which was the focus of the abuse, was destroyed as a good body.
- Hostility permeated her relationships with significant others.

A study by Tucker (1983) of 28 sexually abused young people in Louis-ville, Kentucky revealed that one-quarter of the children actually attempt-ed suicide. This suggests that psychic pain as well as the sexually abused victim's engendered hostility and persecutory guilt makes the young person self-destructive. There is an increased risk of suicide if disclosure work is commenced *before* the young person and the therapist develop a trusting relationship, to contain the range of intense emotions during the disclosure work. *Without a secure relationship* with a therapist and the capacity to mentalize, the young person is very apt to punish herself either during or after the disclosures of sexual abuse for the 'sin' she believes herself to have committed. She suffers a fundamental lack of self-worth, self-respect and self-confidence and feels undeserving of emotional, physical and material satisfaction.

Parental violence and suicide attempts

The young person's despair, hopelessness, and severe self-punitive respon-ses seem linked to the level of parental violence present in the family. Self-destructive behaviour of the children was precipitated by either par-ental beating or a threatened or actual loss of a parent who kills himself. Green (1978) proposed that abused children attempt to escape from their intolerable circumstances by means of suicidal behaviour which usually occurs after an abusive episode. Also the young person's rage against *internalized significant others* can be directed to the self in identification with them.

A severely conflicted marital relationship

Often when couples are in conflict they project their destructive feelings onto the child, who feels a safe target because the child will not divorce them. Intense anger and intense dependency are present in these conflicted rela-tionships. A young person being angered and threatened by a possible loss of one of the parents may attempt suicide.

Neglect

Parental neglect also leaves child with very little sense of self-worth. Lack of internalization of a good enough nurturing object makes the young person feel she doesn't exist and doesn't deserve to exist. The Rey (1994) questions lend further understanding to the young person's internalized and external relationships fostering the suicidal impulse.

Assessment of suicidal risk

Assessment questions for all young people referred for psychological assistance

In any routine assessment of a young person requiring therapy, it is essential to ask certain questions relating to turning for help, self-harm and suicidal thoughts. These questions include:

- What would you do in a time of conflict and difficulty?
- Would you turn to anyone? (If the answer is no, the clinician should be worried that the young person might turn to destructive omnipotence.) If yes, who?
- Have you ever thought of harming yourself?
- Have you ever harmed yourself?

Assessment procedure for a young person who is self-harming and/or is suicidal

If the young person describes thoughts of self-harm or has actually harmed the self then the clinician must ask for further details such as:

- Can you say what particularly was happening to precipitate the self-harm?
- What harm did you actually do and when?
- Have you made any specific plans for harming or killing yourself?
- What has stopped you from fulfilling your plans?
- Might we think together of other ways of looking at resolving the conflict?

If the information received by the clinician concerns current suicidal ideation, then it is essential to work with the young person to share the information with a psychiatrist and with an understanding person in the family and school. If the young person is under the age of 18, the young person must be encouraged to meet the parents/caregivers with the therapist to discuss risks implied by the suicidal plans and motivation. When self-harm or suicide is a distinct possibility a more detailed assessment, asking Dr Rey's (1994) questions described previously and using Litman's (1980) understanding of risks shown in dreams (described below) should occur both during initial assessments and during ongoing treatment. A psychiatrist should be involved in considering whether more intensive therapy, family therapy and/or hospitalization should be undertaken. Most importantly, conditions should be in place for the young person to be safe in relation to her destructive impulses. This may involve obtaining assistance from the police, social services, and/or a family member.

When a serious suicide risk arises in the course of ongoing psychotherapy, similar actions are necessary. The young person should also be given one or more emergency numbers to call. This should be accompanied with the suggestion that in times of extreme distress the young person could call at any time of day or night. Also, the young person could be asked, 'If you decide suicide, would you please promise to call me and speak with me first to let me know what you are intending.' The psychotherapist cannot actually control the young person, but should be doing all that is possible to help ensure that the young person is protected and is empowered to rally her forces tending towards survival (Malan, 1997). Another method is to make an arrangement that the child may go and see a suitably trained professional in the local hospital's Accident and Emergency Department. The young person is given a special letter, which has also been given to the child and Accident and Emergency Department by one of the hospital's child psychiatrists. This procedure has been known to reduce the number of suicide attempts, perhaps because there is an idea that, when the young person is in a seriously conflicted state, the hospital provides a place of safety.

Assessment procedure for all young people who have attempted suicide

There should be adherence to policies and a systematic assessment protocol such as the British NICE guidelines regarding all young suicidal people who have attempted suicide. Ideally a young person should be seen by a psychiatric team member within 24 hours of the suicidal act. Before letting the young person leave hospital, there is a necessity to provide a further therapeutic assessment of the family's capacity to provide a secure, safe base for the young person. If the family is hostile to the young person who has attempted suicide, it is not safe for the young person to go home until sufficient therapeutic work is done to secure a containing family atmosphere. There is also a need for the network surrounding the young person to remain aware of the risk of denial of death, and to continue to place emphasis on the danger still present to the young person's life. The Maudsley Hospital has ascertained that certain types of therapeutic assessments which help people understand their suicide attempt as a method of solving a conflict and help the person see the potential for other ways to deal with the emotional conflict makes it much more likely that the person will return for a follow-up appointment and further therapeutic work.

Dreams as a means of assessing suicidal risk

In *The Dream in Clinical Practice*, Litman (1980) who worked in depth ana-lysing the dreams of suicidal young people, suggests that a young person rarely commits suicide as an impulsive, unpremeditated act. However, some clinicians believe that suicide acts are frequently impulsive. Usually, the idea of suicide is first considered as a potential avenue of escape from intolerable mental pain. Initially, the idea of suicide is alien and frightening. Other solu-tions to the mental pain are sought and attempted, but when these alter-natives fail, the idea of suicide often becomes more attractive. Suicide can be rehearsed in both phantasy and reality.

In clinical practice, understanding the anorectic young person's dreams and drawings can provide clues to potential suicides before the young person is able to speak about suicidal feelings and act upon them. For this reason, I always look at young people's drawings and dreams during the initial assessment as well as throughout the course of therapy. There are some basic themes in drawings and dreams (Litman, 1980) which can alert the therapist to potential suicidal activity. They include the following examples from anorectic girls:

- Themes of death and dead persons:

  Example: I am burning to death in a house on fire.

- Themes of destruction of the self and other persons:

  Example: I had a horrible dream. I am being fired at by soldiers. I die. Then they die. What is the best way of dying? Fast firing guns is better than dying slowly.

- Images of being trapped and struggling unsuccessfully:

  Example: I am running on the beach being chased by a lion looking like a man with claws. I can't escape.

- Peaceful dreams of taking leave of the world and significant others and going elsewhere:

  Example: The woman is being crushed by a roller coaster, then she walks to a beautiful house in the country and has tea and a long conversation with a friend.

It is important to note that these dreams all involve death and can also include ideation that death involves the Self actually staying alive and going to another better world. The dreams can be used to warn the clinician that the young anorectic person is at risk of killing herself to end all feelings. Self-mutilation is different in that the self-mutilator seeks to feel better (1988, p. 262). Of course, it is essential for the therapist to look at death as a metaphor expressing death of internalized figures and death of part of the personality. In listening to dream reports, fine-tuned clinical judgement relying on use of the countertransference is needed. Discussing the young person's conscious motivations, current conflicts and intents, linked with suicidal ideation in the dream, will help the clinician to differentiate between the young person's aggression that can be symbolized and the young person's aggression that will be acted out.

Implications for therapeutic work with the family

It is essential that therapeutic assistance is given to the family to help them provide support to the self-harming or suicidal young person or person who has attempted suicide. The young person is likely to continue to experience moments of virtually unbearable psychic pain. In these moments, self-destruction can be put forward as a solution to the young person's mind unless the family can assist in providing emotional understanding, more support by being more physically present, resolution of conflicts and alternative solutions. Here are some particularly important considerations for the young person and the psychotherapist.

The family into which the suicidal young person returns needs to be assisted in understanding how the family interactions influence the expression of suicidal tendencies. The young person should not be returning to a sadomasochistic relationship with the family that colludes with her suicidal tendencies. The support systems in which the young person lives needs to be containing and receptive to the patient's anxieties, before the young person can safely return home. It is dangerous to have the young person return home until the family is able to accept rather than deny the suicide attempt. Criticism and rejection of the young person for having performed a shameful, impulsive act create a risk for further self-harming and suicidal actions.

Conclusion

The question commonly asked is, 'Can we prevent suicide?' In many situations we can certainly note that an anorectic young person is at risk of self-harm, in addition to anorexia or suicide, by careful use of our countertransference and the child's transference to us during any time we are with the young person in inpatient or outpatient medical settings or in the hospital's Accident and Emergency Department. The denial of the reality of death, however, can permeate professional and family systems. For this reason, it is essential to see young people who have attempted suicide within 24 hours after the act (Campbell and Hale, 1991). Because denial of death can so easily occur it is also crucial to discuss clinical work with self-harming and suicidal young people with one's colleagues (Laufer, 1984). Parents, general practitioners, teachers and other professionals should always be aware of risk when the anorectic young person has an excess of hate, anger, depression. There is also risk of further harm to the anorectic young person's body when, during times of serious conflict, she does not seem to 'hold the hope' either of turning to a secure compassionate attachment figure or of changing her inner situation.

The careful assessment of dreams, suicidal thoughts and the use of Dr Rey's (1994) penetrating questions will assist in predicting risk and taking appropriate safety measures to support the young person. There is, however, the reality that the destructive inner object beckons or bombards a suicidal young anorectic person during times of disappointment and particularly during moments of serious conflict with or separations from a trusted significant other including the psychotherapist, the treatment team, the parents or a friend.

It is particularly important to plan absences of others significant to the young person (parents/therapists) with sufficient warning work through the emotional complications presented by scheduled separations from therapeutic treatment and, especially, when the young person is leaving the inpatient unit with all her hospital carers including her psychotherapist.

During therapeutic work with a suicidal anorectic young person who feels trapped in despair, it is essential to patiently receive and bear the brunt of the young person's painful emotions. At the same time it is necessary to provide some realistic hope and an adequate, consistent, reliable therapeutic structure. The individual psychotherapist's task is to assist in the development of the young person's capacity for mentalization, to be used instead of relying on self-harm and suicide, as ways of coping with intense emotions of rage, hatred, disappointment, and psychic pain. Anne Sexton (1981), a poet who eventually took her own life, viewed her suicide with the remark, 'I have got to have something to hold onto.' 'The family therapist needs to be the catalyst for building meaningful connections between the young person and her parents, peers, teachers, key members of her social network and involved helping professionals from larger systems' (Selekman, 2006).

In conclusion, I would like to cite Donna Williams (1992), who says in her book *Nobody, Nowhere*:

> As much as one might want to, one cannot save another's spirit. One can only inspire the other's spirit to fight to save itself. Perhaps love can inspire but sometimes people must love you enough to declare war.

Note

1 Extracted from *La Femme de Gilles* by Madeleine Bourdouxhe, translated and with an afterword by Faith Evans (published by Daunt Books in 2014). Last section is extracted from the afterword.

Chapter 7

Pervasive retreat

'I didn't want to die but I had to'

Emaciated, eyes closed to the outside world, she lay on the hospital bed. She refused food and drink and seemed not to notice anything, not even the urine trickling out of her. With her straight dark hair and smooth oval Modigliani face, she looked like a porcelain doll. She was motionless throughout the day and night. When after some time she began to respond, she treated any nurse's touch or word like a mosquito creating a stinging irritation. She looked as though the umbilical cord that held her in life had been broken. There seemed to be no emotional point to her existence.

Yufang's history

Yufang is a 17-year-old girl, the middle of three children from a middle-class Chinese family who recently settled in London. She had passed music exams in China and been accepted for admission to a prestigious London music academy, where she would be studying the cello. Her older brother, aged 19, had been left behind in China, where he was studying engineering. Her younger sister, aged 11, had come with the family to London. Her father was a successful businessman and her mother had been a housewife for most of her adult life.

The family was unable to give a detailed picture of Yufang's developmental history. Perhaps her grandmother, with whom the parents had lived in China, might have had a better sense of Yufang as a child, for Yufang's mother was depressed and Yufang was closer to her grandmother. Apparently Yufang's developmental milestones were normal. Her parents described her at age 16 as being hardworking and popular, with a wide circle of friends. She was close to her older brother, who had been very ill with diabetes throughout his life. This had absorbed much of the mother's anxiety and attention. The father had left the family home to work in Russia for 20 months prior to the family coming to this country to live. This had left the mother feeling very unsupported.

When the family moved to London, Yufang met a Colombian boy in her English language school and she became very fond of him. This was her first boyfriend and when both he and her parents simultaneously made separate

DOI: 10.4324/9781003044970-8

trips away from London, Yufang became ill. During the separation from her grandmother in China, her parents and her boyfriend, Yufang began to imagine hearing her father's voice saying, 'I have had an accident.' Around the same time, Yufang complained that the doll she kept on her bed had eyes that haunted her and she was afraid of it. She was afraid to go to sleep for fear of being attacked by it. At this time she began writing to herself, saying she was stupid and selfish.

At this time Yufang also stopped eating and drinking and talking. Her body developed a waxy 'flexibilitas', which meant that she didn't move her body and it stayed in the same position in which her mother put her for long periods of time. She did not even open her eyes to look at anyone. She did not signal when she needed to urinate or defecate. It became clear that it was necessary to tube-feed Yufang. Yufang was admitted to our hospital three months after her family arrived in London.

At the point of admission, she was in a coma. Her right lung had collapsed completely, her kidneys had stopped functioning, and she needed dextrose transfusions because of hypoglycaemia. She was being fed by nasogastric tube and diagnosed as being in a state of depressive stupor.

A Chinese psychiatrist was asked to see her. At that time he said that Yufang had a lack of self-worth, suicidal ideation, and a strong sense of having done something wrong. She had a psychotic depression according to him, but within the first month of administration of psychotropic drugs he recommended, her condition worsened.

By the end of the early stage of her admission, Yufang was completely mute, lying motionless in bed. She was so pale and lifeless that she seemed nearly dead. I felt the medication had not been helpful, but rather dissolved her coping ego-capacities even further so that she retreated into muteness and lay motionless in bed. Yufang had lost the wish to live and was slowly dying.

In desperation, the psychiatrists gave her ECT (electroconvulsive therapy) which momentarily 'awakened her' but then 12 days after the ECT treatments ended she went back into her closed off state. I suggested that I, a psychoanalytic psychotherapist, see her for six days a week for supportive psychotherapy and requested that the psychiatrists hold off ECT until we saw whether or not a relationship with a therapist would enable Yufang to find a way of living without having to have ECT. I was given six weeks to 'trial' supportive psychoanalytic psychotherapy.

In order to treat Yufang, we needed to find some understanding of where her symptoms and illness had come from. Different members of the team had different approaches to this. Even giving a name to her difficulties was complicated; her disorder had been labelled as 'pervasive refusal syndrome' by the Eating Disorder Team at Great Ormond Street Hospital (Lask et. al., 1991). This name, pervasive refusal, is misleading for Yufang felt 'compelled to die' because she felt helpless in the face of overwhelming distress. Later such a disorder was given the name 'pervasive avoidance withdrawal syndrome'

(PAWS) (Lask et al., 2013). For this reason, I prefer to say simply that 'she did not talk, walk or eat' and note that as the course of therapy progressed, Yufang began to develop varying degrees of volition in relation to the pull towards death which had been used as a solution to her overwhelming distress.

It has been pointed out that a sense of helplessness (Garber and Seligman, 1980) leads to a picture characteristic of post-traumatic stress disorder (PTSD). The features illustrated include numbing of responsiveness, reduced involvement with the external world, pervasively diminished interest in the normal activities of daily life, and severely constricted emotions. As the child makes some progress she makes exaggerated startle responses to irritating encounters with people or noise.

These symptoms, shared by young people with PTSD, prompted our psychiatric team to assume with virtual certainty that such a global avoidant response must certainly be linked with a traumatic event such as physical or sexual abuse or else the witnessing of threats and violence at home. In this working context, it was very difficult to maintain a psychoanalytic stance of not-knowing and being curious about who Yufang was and what her internal and external experiences were. In particular it was difficult to remain open to Yufang's other emotions present under her appearance of a helpless, frightened child, a victim.

Nunn and Thompson (1996) suggest a more complicated understanding of not talking, walking and eating. They maintain that separation anxiety and helplessness is a prominent feature. This is accompanied by social withdrawal and depression. The young person feels, and may be actually experiencing, that it is impossible to control situations relating to health, safety, and happiness within the family. He suggests that hopelessness occurs in these situations and prompts the emergence of the regression to not talking, walking or eating in certain young people. As our psychiatric team was so influenced by those ways of interpreting Yufang's regression, as I said before, it was very difficult to maintain an open mind necessary for psychoanalytic psychotherapy, to just use my countertransference to discover clues to Yufang's unique personality and personal narrative.

Yufang's presentation certainly agreed with the wider team's 'helplessness' conceptualization. Because Yufang looked so weak, helpless and vulnerable, it was difficult to imagine or even notice Yufang having any destructive, jealous, contemptuous, omnipotent impulses that could contribute to the causation or perpetuation of her depression and regression. Intellectually, I was aware that it was impossible to facilitate Yufang's development without ridding myself of the notion of her being a 'helpless victim of hostile external events'. I knew that I needed to experience all of her; yet even when, later on, my supervisor suggested to me that some of Yufang's behaviour, including her tendency to giggle, might be contemptuous, I still found it difficult to accept.

How could I even *dare to think* that she had some destructiveness within her? If she did, would it be cruel and damaging to talk about it? This dilemma highlights some of the difficulties that a different set of conceptualizations can lead to when working within a wider team. For me, as the course of treatment progressed, it became clear that Yufang's central psychic defence was a massive denial of conflictual feelings accompanied by projection of her aggression onto others. This was accompanied by intense fears of real or phantasied persecutory fears of aggression from the external world. This different, psychoanalytic way of perceiving Yufang and her illness derived purely from how I experienced her in therapy. However, the questions that follow from this are twofold: how do you come to such an understanding, and how do you then make full use of this understanding to guide the young person towards health within the context of the team with whom you are working? Or, to put it another way, how can we go about treatment of this rare and life-threatening disorder?

Treatment

My experience of Yufang and other young people with similar difficulties has led me to the understanding that in order to be successful, the treatment approach needs to be both psychotherapeutic and focused on good teamwork, helping both the wider staff team and the parents to understand the psychoanalytic issues as they arise.

At this time there was a popular notion in British child psychiatry that psychoanalytic psychotherapy should be given only after a young person regains her normal weight, for a notion existed that psychotherapy disturbs and pesters a 'very ill' or severely depressed, emaciated young person, rather than helping her. The current child psychiatry texts also referred to psychoanalytic psychotherapy as being suitable mainly for young people who have the capacity to express themselves verbally, use symbolic thought and have little difficulty in forming interpersonal relationships (Graham, 1986). Obviously, I felt differently, and such statements as these prompted me to edit a book, *The Silent Child: Communication Without Words* (Magagna, 2012).

I do not support the idea that young people who do not speak should not be offered a specifically modified form of psychoanalytic psychotherapy, nor do I believe in the notion that one should wait till a young person is physically fit until they have psychotherapy. Although the mind is compromised by severe starvation and physical illness, the young person is terrified to be in this predicament and requires the attentive, empathic thoughtfulness and physical care similar to that of a newborn baby. Without the containing presence of a fully equipped psychotherapist, the young person may never regain the wish to live. I have known of a young person living for ten years in this condition of feeling 'compelled to die' because during those ten years the appropriate psychotherapeutic and psychiatric care to meet her particular specialized needs and those of her family was not found.

One problem is that underneath the symptoms of not talking, not walking, not eating may lay various different psychopathologies including anxiety disorders, anorexia nervosa, psychotic depression, borderline personality disorder, incipient schizophrenia, obsessive compulsive disorder and various phobias. A combination of specifically tailored family psychotherapy, individual psychotherapy and specialized medical and nursing care for a particular young person can result in long term recovery, but someone with incipient schizophrenia will need years of on-going psychotherapy to develop and maintain a reasonable life. I have been involved in providing psychoanalytic psychotherapy or psychotherapy supervision for 18 of these non-speaking young people, both boys and girls, 'compelled to die'. With frequent individual psychotherapy, family therapy and appropriate medical care being provided for 12–18 months most have fully recovered. One exception is a young person who has made enormous progress from a severely regressed state but needs much longer-term psychotherapy for she has schizophrenic symptoms (she is described in Chapter 5).

The psychotherapeutic approach involves work in the transference, looking at the 'here and now' relationship through careful observation of the relationship existing between the young person and the psychotherapist. It also involves a deep contact with the therapist's countertransference experiences, which inform understanding of the non-speaking young person (Racker, 1974). A psychotherapy training involving infant observation (Bick, 1968) allows the psychotherapist to trace the sequence of nonverbal interaction between the young person and the therapist and lend meaning to it, much as a mother does with a non-speaking baby. Most importantly, the focus is on the therapist reaching to the very deepest part of his/her personality to find empathic attunement to the physical and emotional experience of the young person.

With such a very ill young person, initially it is the psychotherapist who needs to make demands on herself to fully understand the present moment with the young person, rather than expecting anything at all from the young person. My experience has led me to believe that the impediments to the young person's psychological progress are threefold: the context to which the young person will return may not be or be felt by the young person to be safe, nurturing, trustworthy and supportive; secondly, the context (including the milieu and therapies in which the young person is participating) may be 'pushing, intrusive and demanding' of the non-speaking young person and thirdly, the staff and/or parents may continue to experience latent or overt aggression towards the young person, who frequently evokes a feeling of impotence in those caring for her.

The secret for therapeutic progress is for the multidisciplinary team to remain very patient while comprehensively understanding and bearing the young person's overwhelming feelings and anxieties about living. At the same time, it is necessary for them to simultaneously work collaboratively and therapeutically with the family to resolve conflictual issues surrounding such an ill, non-speaking and non-eating young person. Of course such a non-talking, walking eating young person needs nutrition and bodily care, but no demands should be put on the young person to speak. The young person will speak when feeling safe and trusting while experiencing being empathically and deeply understood.

Therapeutic work involves careful attention to the total contextual milieu and particular attention must be given to the splitting off and projection of undesirable feelings to staff, parents or the young person. A great deal of mutual blaming can occur when all parties involved feel impotent to immediately facilitate the child's significant improvement. The therapeutic work involves family therapy, parental counselling, and a coordinated multidisciplinary team, including a psychiatrist, individual and family psychotherapists, a physiotherapist, a teacher and nurses, who meet regularly to think about their collaborative efforts. The parents are considered to be therapeutic agents working alongside the multidisciplinary team to promote a nurturing and facilitating environment for their child.

So far it feels very straightforward. But how does one apply these principles in practice? I will now share with you some examples from our work with Yufang, looking at both the teamwork that was necessary to support her and her family and the psychoanalytic psychotherapy that helped her to develop the capacity to think about emotional experiences and resolve conflicts on the basis of thoughtful processing of interpersonal events.

Milieu treatment: working with the team to help Yufang

A coordinated system involving family and staff surrounding the child was essential. Each day I would meet the paediatric nurses to discuss their experiences with Yufang. They felt totally bewildered by a young person whom they felt was unresponsive and, later, hostile to any gesture of concern or practical care that they offered her. She made them feel impotent in using their usual nursing skills and this prompted some hostility and lack of warmth on their part. I encouraged the nurses to understand that, although she wasn't speaking to them or responding warmly to them, they didn't mean that she wouldn't appreciate being understood and nurtured in a non-intrusive way by them. She wouldn't eat, but she might listen if they played soothing music to her, for she was a musician after all. She didn't open her eyes much, but she could listen to stories that they might tell her from a book or from their experiences of the day. I indicated that I was not really indicating that they were to do something strange and reminded them that a mother generally spends 12 months with her young baby, caring for the baby and speaking to the baby about many things without expecting that the baby respond to the mother through speaking. The mother and baby are learning to understand one another. I warned the nurses that their task would be made more difficult if they expected a response from Yufang, because that would be experienced as 'pushing her' and making intrusive demands on her rather than understanding and supporting her in this state of regression.

Gradually, after the nurses had sufficient support during regular times to share some of their frustrations and sense of rejection by Yufang, they became interested in the task of nurturing her. They compassionately related to her with their thoughts, their singing, their music, their showing her pictures and their reading to her until she developed sufficient hope again to respond to people. I encouraged them to feel what it must be like to be her in order to stay attuned to her. I also encouraged the nurses to talk with her about not-too-personal thoughts about the day on the ward, or life outdoors, which could be seen from the window. I also suggested that the nurses think of creating a dialogue between what they put into words and feelings and Yufang's response to what they offered her. I gave them examples of how they might comment on how she was moving away from them with a flinch or moving towards them with a quick glance. The nurses were encouraged to use their intuition to describe the different emotional meanings of Yufang moving towards them or pulling away from them. For example, they might say, 'You are looking at me, trying to find out just what kind of person I am', or 'I seem to be frightening you' or 'I seem to be making you annoyed with me'. I encouraged Yufang's mother to approach Yufang similarly while sharing news from home and news from Yufang's brother and grandmother who lived in China.

I encouraged the nurses to stop talking to me 'about Yufang' and to describe the process of interaction between her and them, thinking about how they and she were developing a relationship in which she spoke through gesture and they responded with empathic feeling, identifying with her, and then giving meaning to her actions. The discussion was now no longer focused on Yufang's symptoms but rather on how both the nurses and Yufang were relating and how the nurses were developing their skills of understanding their emotional responses to her and her emotional responses to them. For example, a nurse reported she said, 'Yufang, I've brought a book for you I thought you might like.' The nurse would open the book, talk about some of the pictures in the book, and then, noticing Yufang's immobility, the nurse, not being able to avoid feeling rejected, would say, 'You don't seem to feel that I have brought you something of any interest to you.' On another occasion a nurse said, 'I'd like to read you a little bit of a story about leaving one's country of origin,' and then, seeing Yufang look up momentarily, the nurse said, 'You seem to like my talking about people who have left their country.'

The nurses no longer felt impotent, rather they felt challenged by this idea of relating to Yufang as a mother would to a young infant, interpreting the young person's nonverbal relationship with her. Unfortunately, so much of the time, there was a painful contrast between other young people on the ward, who were friendly and responsive, and unresponsive Yufang, who was often regressed and in 'her own world'.

I had to spend a lot of time helping the nurses to think they were nurturing a little hope in Yufang and it would take a long time to see any visible sign of what was growing inside her. I also suggested that Yufang's non-responsiveness could also possibly be a protection against disappointment. If she hoped for something, she might be hurt and disappointed. If no one and no act mattered, she would never feel disappointed, no longer feel pain again. In this way I tried to help the nurses realize that they would need to support each other as they felt so rejected and disappointed with Yufang's slow progress. I affirmed that, even if they did not see Yufang make progress, they should not feel they were useless in their attempt to foster her wish to be alive. Patience was an essential ingredient to helping Yufang and when this was not present and Yufang was pressured in anyway, she regressed. I also lightly mentioned that being rejected by a young person can stir up other feelings of rejection and resulting resentment, which might not be directly the result of Yufang's rejection of them.

The nurses and I gradually shared a perception that Yufang could receive their concern, their understanding without showing if she has accepted it or felt it to be helpful. We talked about the defensive part of Yufang... but how there might be a hidden child part knowing, receiving, feeling grateful to be understood. I shared with the nurses my sense that we were working towards understanding Yufang... and that was her only hope of survival! I said we had no reason to believe that Yufang would not gradually respond to their nurturing, empathic understanding. I encouraged them to hold onto patience and hope for a better relationship with Yufang in the future.

As much as possible I was talking about developing a relationship with Yufang, observing her responses to them through her eyes, hands, mouth, body posture and understanding their particular feelings in their relationship with Yufang, rather than focusing on 'what Yufang was doing'. The focus was on empathically observing a process of interaction and discovering its meaning for both Yufang and the nurses.

Joined-up teamwork: creating a therapeutic space in which to work

As I reflected on this first period of Yufang's hospitalization, I began questioning my aims as a psychotherapist. Why was it that I felt so determined to rescue Yufang? I was struck by the readiness with which I became angry or critical of the psychiatrists, the mother, and the nurses. It was much easier to be critical than to face my own incapacities and lack of understanding in this formidable task of working with Yufang. It was also much easier to split off and project my own aggression, my own violent phantasies, into the ECT and the two psychiatrists recommending it, while owning my own loving, caring feelings towards Yufang. It also seemed to bring a kind of inner psychological relief to locate aggression in others rather than in Yufang, a hopeless, ill and potentially dying young person.

Splitting of love and hate, projection of aggression into others, seemed to be an accompaniment to the multidisciplinary team's work with Yufang. We needed to acknowledge and integrate these feelings within ourselves to be able to deeply understand who Yufang was and the nature of our relationship with her. For Yufang, I was part of a clinic team, partnered with the family therapist, and the psychiatrist managing the treatment. When Yufang met me, she rubbed her hands, looked at the black-and-blue marks on them and fostered my temptation to become cocooned with her against the hostile external world that had given her pre-treatment medication marks linked with the ECT which I was against. In this frame of mind, I became too protective, too maternal. The tone of my voice was too soothing. It lacked sufficient strength and thoughtfulness. In order for me to find the appropriate therapeutic relationship with Yufang, it was necessary for me to acknowledge that I had been part of the therapeutic team that had permitted ECT to take place. This was working in the total transference espoused by psychoanalyst Betty Joseph (1985, 557–453) and described in 'Psychodynamic psychotherapy in an inpatient unit' (Magagna, 1998).

I also had to accept that I could not evade my disquiet and guilt regarding my aggression by evacuating it into external figures. I knew that it was essential to be linked in a collaborative way with the psychiatrists and others in order to maintain a therapeutic space for thinking about the team and family dynamics surrounding Yufang's individual psychotherapy. It would be confusing for all concerned if we did not have a 'joined-up' approach and the continuation of the psychotherapy and development of my capacity as a psychotherapist were dependent on reintegrating my projections and helping the team contain projections surrounding work with Yufang.

As the weeks passed, the nurses and I became aware of how much we expected some response from Yufang, rationally knowing that we should be simply providing deeply compassionate understanding to Yufang and our feelings in being with her. Each day I listened to the nurses and shared comments relating to the slightest responsiveness from her. 'She looked interested in the music!' 'She cried, she looked at me today!' There were days on end when Yufang simply lay in bed not moving, when it was easy to feel irritation or even anger with her for 'not trying' as though she were completely competent to challenge her severely regressed psychological condition. Then we had to step back and mentor our own interactions with Yufang... what did we do which fostered an appreciative look and what did we do which pushed her back into retreat?

For example, on one occasion the music teacher managed to get Yufang to sit in a chair with a cello between her legs. This was obviously far too advanced for her, but when he felt disappointed with Yufang's failure to lift her hand to the cello, the music teacher immediately became a persecutory figure from whom she turned away. The cello became 'a bad object', although Yufang had loved music from the time she began playing instruments at the age of five. We learned not to take independent moves without checking out with each other whether or not we were 'moving too fast forward'.

We clarified our therapeutic aims for the team: our task was to create a therapeutic space for thinking about how Yufang felt in her relationships with us each day. We needed structure to the day with nurturing experiences for her, offers of music, stories, conversation and thinking about how she interacted with us. We were not to create expectations of her, for if we did she perceived us as horrible demanding figures. We could think of minimal structured progressions in the structure of activities provided for Yufang and we needed to think together about the ways in which we encouraged her development.

Our responses to Yufang, our countertransference, had to be carefully monitored and discussed. Yufang's withdrawn state could leave us feeling hurt and deprived by her! Yufang's role as a patient was in danger of being compressed into the gratification of our need to feel helpful and not destructive in our roles as nurses and therapists. Our frustration and sense of impotence led us to detect that in many of our comments there was a sense of superiority, barely perceptible, but present, as we professionals searched for and discussed weaknesses in Yufang's family. A tone of blame and irritation in our comments about the family concealed the team members' annoyance with each other's differing points of view about how to proceed and about what was being experienced by Yufang. Our comments included many hypotheses about the damage that may have been done to Yufang by her family and by her boyfriend who had left her to go on holiday.

Present in the team dynamics seemed to be a thwarted desire to be angry with someone: the father, the family, the doctor, the referring psychiatrist. The theme of 'who is to blame' seemed to permeate the team's informal discussions. Scorn was barely concealed – why had the doctor let things go on so badly for so long? Why did he let her get so emaciated before referring her? Why did he pump her with chlorpromazine, whose side-effect made her considerably more stuporous? This attempt to place blame somewhere was shared by the family. They were impatient with our lack of progress and lack of certainty about a healthy future for Yufang. Why hadn't we given her the right medication? We didn't seem to be making her better – rather, they felt we were hurting her for she was beginning to cry, something which she had rarely done before!

To make very critical remarks amongst ourselves and about each other seemed an easy, common outlet for our ignorance and impotence – experiences shared by the treatment team and the family. Blaming also defended us against experiencing Yufang's deep despair and our despair in being unable to readily relieve her of her psychic pain. Blaming also interfered with a deeper exploration of our own internal psychological states and the team dynamics involving revived old sibling rivalries. At times we also competed with each other as to who had been most helpful to Yufang. All these issues could only be understood, not through textbooks, but through patient curiosity in our exploration of loving and hating feelings existing in Yufang, the family and the multidisciplinary team working together with the family.

In retrospect, I realized that blaming the family was preventing us from looking at the hostility present in Yufang's relationships with her family and us. The professional network was in fact unwittingly re-enacting an unconscious process, not yet understood, within the family dynamics (Britton, 1989). It was more difficult to create 'a containing treatment framework' for bearing paranoid anxieties and living with Yufang's despair and hidden hostility projected into us. Blaming had a certain energy but what we needed was courage to sustain the painful hope that if we could nurture Yufang with our understanding of her feelings, she might be drawn to life, to a figure who understands and provides hope for life. We worried that sustaining hope would be futile, for Yufang seemed very attached to a 'death-wish', to a sense that there was 'no point in living'.

The family met weekly with a psychotherapist to assist in the task of supporting Yufang and developing insight into the family interactions that might interfere with or support her progress. When Yufang was able to sit in a chair, she joined the family meetings, even though she was mute and withdrawn. During these sessions the family members each shared worries about Yufang and what they felt it was like 'to be in her shoes'. The family tried to find ways of supporting Yufang and each other during this family crisis. They also talked about their deep sense of loss of the grandmother, their son, their home, their Chinese customs, language and food. Everything was so different for each of them. The mother also described how she also worried about the life of their oldest boy, aged 19, who suffered from a severe diabetic condition with which he sometimes went into a coma. The entire family was sad about separation from all that was familiar and a source of comfort security and happiness in their lives.

Yufang seemed to hold the extreme version of the family's reluctance to take in, feel, and accept the sadness and resentment about separation from all things loved and familiar. The family had borne the separation from father for 20 months and had little control over father's unilateral decision that the family was moving to London. Each family member, particularly the mother, felt the need to passively accept the transition to London in order not to lose the father on a more permanent basis. The father and mother were unable to take into account the adverse emotional aspects of moving to London without the English language to smooth their entry. Work with the family helped contain their anxieties; they became more able to allow themselves to own their own sad and conflicting feelings previously projected into Yufang, and to support Yufang in her individual psychotherapy. It is a matter of some controversy, but as demonstrated in Yufang's family, the symptom bearer maybe be holding shared family defences against psychic pain and thus require family therapy and/or parental counselling accompanying the individual psychotherapy for one young person. I feel that family therapy is essential in ensuring the young person's on-going therapeutic progress beyond hospitalization.

While offering Yufang psychotherapy six times a week, I also engaged the nurses and Yufang's mother in containing Yufang's emotional experiences. Initially they had talked about her feeling in a 'not good, not safe' new place. Later they began talking about her need to find a safe place in hospital with them. Then they were able to describe split emotions: being curled up in bed felt good, but being outside bed felt bad. Gradually more positive experiences were able to be described to her: the nurses were able to say that Yufang was pleased when her mother was with her, pleased when the nurse was present. She looked forward to her mother's return and her favourite nurses being on a shift. The nurses and mother were encouraged to inform Yufang about when they would be away and when they would be returning. They then were encouraged to describe in detail to her when she felt distressed or angry because they were late, were away, were talking to others, or had misunderstood what she experienced. The nurses and her mother were also encouraged to comment upon when Yufang liked an experience and when she was annoyed by silence or too much talk. Mother's and the nurses' giving words to her experiences gradually enabled Yufang to find her own voice and speak about her own feelings.

Individual psychotherapy

During the initial part of our work together, Yufang had her eyes closed, did not speak and in any case, barely knew English. In fact, neither Yufang nor her mother spoke English very well, and for this reason Yufang had been studying English during the first three months in this country. It wasn't clear during conversations whether she was simply not thinking or not understanding my English... or both. If she spoke at all, she certainly did not show a wish for a personal relationship.

My own personal task in working with Yufang were similar in many respects to that of the parents and other members of the multidisciplinary team. I needed to be attuned to my emotional and physical experience of being with Yufang in the present moment of the session in order to give meaning to her communications, which involved many feelings being projected onto me and transmitted in a nonverbal way. This work is similar to that described by Schore (2002). Yufang's confusion and lack of integration could be linked to a mismatch in communication in her primary experience as a baby with her parents. For this reason she needed me to consider her primitive experiences in her regressed state, including sensations and the movement or stillness of her body, before she could symbolize these experiences and put them into dreams or drawings or words. An integration of her body and psychological self could then occur. Deep inside, Yufang was hungry for us to comprehend her, even though initially she seemed cocooned with mouth closed to food, eyes closed to people, words unavailable to share her feelings. Walking in the world was given up in favour of residing in some form of womb-like claustrum (Meltzer, 1992) where no thinking was present.

Psychotherapy is only partly a talking cure, for that which cannot be conceptualized or spoken about by the young person can nevertheless be conveyed emotionally and physically when present with the therapist. I attempted to create a narrative of Yufang's experiences through describing shared, obvious, external family issues such as the loss of the grandmother, the brother and homeland and the frightening anger of father's and mother's that at times left Yufang feeling without helpful parents. I also described some problem she had in relation to the Colombian boyfriend without being clear exactly what had been upsetting about the relationship apart from his leaving her for two weeks to go to Colombia to visit his family. My real task, though, was to help Yufang note her present emotional experiences with me and lend thought to them in order that they would not be so overwhelming to her.

Silence as deprivation or communion

There were other issues I had to take into account in my approach to working with Yufang. I did not think it was helpful for Yufang to come into the room and sit in a motionless, severely depressed silence for more than five minutes. My impression was that if I did stay silent, she felt I had invited her to be in a room to be deprived of my attempts to nurture her through sharing my thoughts and feelings with her. I thought being silent would be like a mother not talking to her infant, not treating her infant as a baby with a mind. At other times there existed between Yufang and me a prevailing desire for a static space devoid of feelings, because feelings were so disturbing to her. Hospital staff had tried asking questions but Yufang had remained with her lips shut most of the time. My own questions took the form of being curious aloud *to myself* in Yufang's presence. I sometimes talked to a stuffed animal which I had in the room, describing our experience together. I used various ways of thinking aloud to myself, for questions and thoughts about Yufang that were directed to Yufang could very easily be experienced as intrusive and demanding.

What seemed most important was my talking about Yufang's experience at that moment in the room and generating in her an interest in her emotional life. I tried to identify with Yufang, using her physical posture, glance of her eye, expression of her mouth and hands, to describe what she was feeling when with me and how she was responding to what I said. At times I spoke in first person as though I were Yufang in various developmental stages. Holding a small doll, I would 'be Yufang' as a younger child and then talk to Yufang the older child doll about this 'younger regressed person'. Often I described things as I would to a very young child, talking about what Yufang and those around her had been doing during the day, talking about how she responded to her mother coming and staying on the paediatric ward and going away from her. Then I would think in more detail about the experiences that Yufang had. She lacked the capacity to observe herself but observations were provided by the staff's daily descriptions of their mutual interactions with Yufang. These observations of how Yufang greeted a particular staff member, how she responded to the staff member, including me, talking to her, reading to her, leaving her were all part of my on-going dialogue with Yufang.

Meanwhile, the focus of my thinking was on the developing relationship present at that moment between 'the-little-child' in Yufang and me. I described a mood that I felt in the room on each given day: 'good to be here together', 'suspicious of me', 'curious about what I will say', 'pushing me away'. I might comment on how she greeted me when I first met her that new day. Each nonverbal response that Yufang made became her having a dialogue with me and provided a possible opportunity for me to think and speak with her. For example, I would say: 'You looked up when I came into the room. You have been looking into my eyes listening with interest some of the time I have been speaking. Now, when we part, I know you can nod goodbye, but you have chosen not to.' Yufang giggled when I said this. I then said, 'You giggled as though you agreed that you could have nodded goodbye. Perhaps I should experience "the goodbye".'

My aim was to meet Yufang's most immediate emotions present in the therapy. This involved 'listening to her mood' as one listens to music. I thought if she were playing her cello for me her music would go where her words were not able to go and then I might understand more… but that was for later. Now, as Yufang remained immobile, I had to allow her mood to enter me and then I named it. My idea was that internal change in Yufang could best be facilitated through comments that met her feelings and anxieties in the immediate present in our encounter. When Yufang subsequently used words, I would rely on her to talk about whatever was on her mind, as I would with any other person in psychotherapy. In the initial phase, however, Yufang was primarily lifeless, mute and as there was no verbal conversation, it seemed necessary for me to use my heart, my body, my soul to help her gather her *whole being* together to be emotionally present; in the room. I sometimes experienced an image of a turtle gradually peeping out of an impermeable shell and disappearing back inside the darkness. I told stories of turtles, snails, possum and children developing hope and courage. Sometimes I even used part of a poem or story book with pictures which I spontaneously recounted in my own words. My feeling emotionally present and using words of understanding were vital in evoking Yufang's desire to leave the dark world of 'not-thinking' and find and use her apparently disintegrated emotional and mental functioning again.

Using dolls for stories of the young person's experiences

I sometimes brought out a set of dolls and told stories to Yufang about her relationships with different members in her family including her absent grandmother and older brother. For example, I used the dolls to dramatize the story of how Yufang's mother came to visit her daughter and how for a moment they greeted each other, looking at one another and how her mother fed her soup. (Although Yufang still had the nasogastric tube, she had begun accepting being fed by spoon if her mother was doing the feeding.) Initially, I told the story in the third person, more emotionally distant, sitting slightly to the side of Yufang. I was deliberately leaving her free to ignore all that I was saying. Occasionally Yufang looked at or touched one of the family dolls that she wanted me to think about and I would say something about that person, telling her about what I know about her relationship with that member of her family. I would describe that person. Although she was actually 17, when Yufang was more regressed it was easier to use toy animals to tell stories about her life on the ward. I talked about the frightened rabbit, 'very alert to sound', 'closing her eyes', 'wanting to run away from everyone and everything that touched her heart'.

Later on in therapy, however, I spoke more directly to Yufang. For example, when she touched the father doll, I said, 'You seem very frightened of your father. He is "the boss" of the family and sometimes he becomes very angry, and you didn't know what in the world to do then.' Yufang was quiet and subsequently tears rolled down her face as she cried silently. She made no effort to wipe the tears away. At another time, when she touched the mother doll, I said, 'Your mother seems so loving to you, but so sad. She also seems frightened of your father and feels she absolutely must obey him.' In response, Yufang stiffened and then remained immobile, not looking up. On another occasions, I used the dolls to show the whole family crying. I said, 'Your parents, but particularly your mother, are sad about being in this new country with a different language, sad to have left your brother behind in China.' Yufang looked at me and I said, 'You need the protection of your mother and me in hospital. Now you are beginning to accept us.'

Within this framework of enacting family issues through play, I was able to comment on my sense of our transference relationship, at times a confusing experience in which Yufang distrusted me as a frightening figure and at times moments in which Yufang depended on me as a nurturing figure, one who was curious about her experiences and trying to understand them with her. Part of the success of this therapy was due to our very frequent, but half-hour meetings, allowing us to keep the scattered shifting view of me and others in mind within a steady, emotionally containing context.

Illustrations of the individual psychotherapeutic work as it progressed.

As this chapter comes to a close, I would like to illustrate some particularly difficult aspects of my dialogue with Yufang, using my countertransference to her nonverbalized cues as a focus for my communication with her. I shall draw on sequential selections from our sessions during the psychotherapy and subsequently discuss them.

Initially Yufang seemed to have little awareness of many fragmented parts of her personality which were isolated, lonely and out of communication with everyone including herself. There was very little sense of a Self present. Following the technique recommended by Rosenfeld (1987b) I began the psychotherapy on six days per week. The sessions were shortened to half an hour because Yufang was initially too weak, too tired to maintain a focus for longer. Initially she remained verbally mute, immobile, with an incredibly sad, vacant look on her face. The following session, typical of the early sessions, is from the second week of Yufang's therapy.

When I greet her with a friendly hello, Yufang's eyes remain turned downwards into her lap. I physically experience my 'hello' dropping to the ground. She holds onto my arm with much of her weight resting upon me as we go to the therapy room. She walks very slowly, shuffling her feet along the shiny hospital floor. Yufang closes her eyes completely as she sits down, but I can tell that she is listening to the irregular banging sound of the malfunctioning radiator. Yufang begins to show tension and fear in her face. Opening her eyes, she searches for the door. I say, 'This room doesn't feel good. The sounds are disturbing. You don't like them. You want to get out. You don't like my speaking either.' I say this avoiding looking directly at Yufang for fear I shall be experienced as too intrusive, but when I do look at her briefly, she looks into my eyes for a second. I think she felt understood by me. As Yufang glances down at her feet again she struggles unsuccessfully to mouth the word, 'Go'. I speak as though I am Yufang saying in a frightened but insistent tone, 'Let me go. I don't want to be here!' After a few moments Yufang, almost imperceptibly, nods in agreement. I say then, 'You are so uncertain about what any sound means. You aren't certain if I can be trusted to keep you safe in this room, this room, which isn't your usual place, which is your bed.' In response Yufang glances briefly at me.

I am aware that making changes is frightening to Yufang. Leaving her bed seems to create a sense of being thrust out into a dangerous, hostile world in which anything can happen. I understand that Yufang was not only disturbed by the new space, by the sound of a broken ventilator, she also wanted to get out of my room, out of my presence.

Yufang at times viewed me as a dangerous enemy threatening to break into her protective shell of non-feeling, of depersonalization, of non-thinking. Yufang seemed encapsulated, like children Spitz (1965) described, or like the Jewish refugee orphans who, having no emotional link with anyone, give themselves up to death. However, for a moment, Yufang was able to meet me with fleeting acknowledgement that I existed and that I understood how frightened she felt. She had come alive to her feeling of fear and that was better than not knowing what she felt.

It was only much later that Yufang let me know that there was a malevolent force, a voice in her head condemning her to starve and to die. This sense of being a passive victim of imposed cruelty is a major problem in non-speaking and non-eating young people. Nine months into therapy, Yufang told me about the beginning of her illness: 'When I was ill I had to starve myself. I had to die. I didn't want to die, but I had to. I starved and became unconscious. I felt I was dead.' Yufang also explained some of the pressure towards retreating even further into a shell of 'not-knowing':

> When I was ill, I could not look in a mirror. I could not look in a mirror because I did not know who I saw. I could not see myself. I saw another girl. I thought I was someone else. I felt I was a girl, my friend, who had difficulties with her parents. I felt strange when I couldn't see myself in the mirror. I worried about other children looking at me, because I was afraid that they could see through me.

Yufang was describing how she had lost a sense of her *Self*. She did not feel her ordinary Self, but was depersonalized. She was passively experiencing herself as under instructions from a malevolent, destructive part of her personality which she did not experience as part of herself. This split-off destructive part dictated how she must treat her *Self*; moreover, she felt she had no *Self* available to struggle with 'the dictator'. Yufang movingly said, 'I didn't *want* to die, but I *had* to.'

Now a further series of illustrations from eight sessions will show how I attempted to use Yufang's communications to elucidate her relationship to the internal parental figures as represented by me in the transference relationship. It was through a detailed experience of the transference that I was able to assist Yufang in deepening her understanding of the conflicts in her relationships with internalized parents and siblings. Lending thought to feelings somehow enabled Yufang to develop an internal psychic structure able to bear the stresses of her external life. Through her more developed internal psychic structure she found the courage to move from her regressed state of not talking, walking or eating. I was also able to gain more comprehension of internal and external factors contributing to Yufang's depression and regression.

Another second-week session

Yufang is not speaking, but her fingers are picking away at the skin of her thumb in a very aggressive way. She stops moving her hands, becomes completely motionless apart from her eyes which guard my eyes attentively. I suggest, 'You look at me wondering what I am thinking about your picking. Can I accept your picking?'

In the following session of the same week, Yufang's eyelids begin to flicker as she initiates a tumultuous, unrelenting sobbing. I feel the convulsion of sadness erupting from her.

A fifth-week session

As she wanders into the session, Yufang sways precariously, stepping from foot to foot, as she tries to lift each foot. She cannot seem to find her balance and feels like a toddler requiring support as she is beginning to walk. I know Yufang is not under the effect of any drugs or medication, but her giggling makes it look as if she is drunk without much of a thinking-self present. After she has collected herself in the chair, she does not speak for about 15 minutes of the session. I make some comments and subsequently Yufang says, 'Dream about brother.' She then begins sobbing with a very painful grimace. She says, 'No more,' but she is reluctant to leave. I say, 'I am needed to hold your sobbing self. You don't want to go out and be sad without me.'

In a session later that week, she says 'brother dead', 'must die'. I suggest, 'Your brother feels dead. You don't see him. You feel now you must die.' I think she is implying that she must die because she has killed her brother in her dream and she isn't sure if it is a dream from her internal reality or a fact from external reality.

A sixth-week session

Yufang spends the whole week with a pain in her leg, with no apparent underlying physical difficulty. She is virtually unable to walk to the session, but with much encouragement and help she comes. I talk about: 'Poor leg. It is feeling so much pain. It is suffering a hurt from somewhere.' As I speak, Yufang's still statue-like face unfolds from being expressionless to being contorted with pain, with her eyelids flickering rapidly as tears flow down her face. Her nose is also dripping. As usual she makes no effort to wipe her nose or her face, which is covered in tears. After a few moments, I offer her a tissue which she does not acknowledge or accept. Instead, Yufang bites her lip, then looks into my eyes and opens her mouth, but no sounds emerge. She turns her head away from me. I say, 'You want me to know something very important that makes you cry. You feel you are not allowed or you do not dare to tell me.' When it is time to leave the room, Yufang hangs onto my arm, and she will not let go when I leave her at her bedside. It takes some moments of saying, 'I will come back to see you, but it is very hard to say goodbye. It is hard to be left with all these feelings with which you want me to help you.'

The day after this session, Yufang is playing her cello for the first time since she became ill. I heard some of her playing which went on continuously for five hours. The music was monotonous, not melodic, and not reflective of any of Yufang's previous considerable musical skills. It was more like sawing out one or two tones in a grating, irritating way. Her lips had not opened much to speak, but now Yufang was finding some way of expressing the discordant, irritating feelings present while with me and during the separation from me.

Yufang could not bear to tear herself away from the cello either and finally the nurses managed to struggle with her to leave it aside and rest.

A seventh-week session

For the first time ever, Yufang arrives looking somewhat cheerful as though the sun has come out after a flooding rain. She doesn't speak. She appears bored with me and she yawns while I am talking with her. In fact, Yufang appears to be completely out of touch with the fact that I am in the room with her. After I have spoken for some time, Yufang silently mouths some words, yawns, goes blank. This is very disconcerting, for she is emotionally present one moment and then mentally absent. I speak a little more, 'You seem to just fall into sleep, cover your mind, not let me touch your heart. Then for an instant you join me. Then you leave me again.' Yufang moves her lips again without looking at me and begins to cough. She coughs several times. She seems to almost fall backwards as she gets up to walk out of the session. When I put my arm out to hold her, she leans back on me as though she is going to collapse completely into me. After this session, Yufang virtually stopped drinking and eating for four days. She also did not utter a word to anyone including her mother.

Comments on the second to seventh week

The narrative of Yufang's inner life experiences was beginning to be repeated in her transference relationship to me. In the second session when Yufang picked her finger, I commented that she was punishing herself or someone in her mind, perhaps me. I felt that the picking of her finger was linked with an attack on an internalized figure. Later her fingers were very red from her scratching skin off them and I described what she was doing. At this moment Yufang categorically denied that she was picking. She was not able to accept any responsibility for any angry or destructive impulses.

During the fifth week, although she said she didn't remember dreams, she was able to remember a dream of an important relationship with her brother. In the dream he was dead. It felt premature to interpret my sense that her developing closeness to her mother and me meant that she wanted to push her brother out of her mother's mind. I could, however, interpret that as she grew more trusting of me, she wanted to push the *other young people* out of my mind. Her punishment was that she should die in identification with the 'dead internal brother' represented by the attacked 'other young people' whom I saw for psychotherapy.

Separations were difficult in themselves, but each separation evoked unworked-through feelings about previous separations, which included feeling left by her mother who remained severely depressed as well as very pre-occupied by the unstable diabetic problems of the older brother who remained in China; separation from her grandmother in China who had previously replaced her mother as her prime caregiver; separation from the Colombian language school boyfriend whose unknown relationship with her and his departure might have precipitated her breakdown into her psychotic depression, not talking, walking or eating. Yufang's growing wish to possess her mother more completely for herself and her growing trust in me left her feeling overwhelmed with possessive jealousy.

In the second and sixth week of psychotherapy Yufang goes deep within herself to experience a multitude of different emotions which erupt in a convulsion of tears. In the sixth week she attempts to give these emotions words to share with me, but there is a 'biting her lip', a holding her lip shut, as though she feels too worried to open herself to knowing her inner experiences more fully. Because her emerging but previously denied feelings are too overwhelming, there is a fear they will take her over. I also wonder if she is 'forbidden to speak' by a part of herself, or maybe even by others.

Yufang's primitive protections against knowing her overwhelming painful feelings lead to somatization of psychic pain in her leg and picking, which creates physical pain, which is less intense than emotional pain. She also becomes mentally blank and enters a dissociated state, somatizing through yawning, coughing, losing muscle control of her body and not being able to walk, not drinking, eating or talking for four days. Later Yufang used her cello playing both to express the unspeakable unpleasant feelings and to 'hold herself together' emotionally through non-stop playing until the nurses stopped her. Yufang may have found some relief in pouring out 'sounds of feelings' expressed through the grinding monotonous music that entered all of us who were listening. Within seven weeks, the narrative or Yufang's inner life revealed dependence, pain of loss, anger about loss, hostile feelings and persecutory anxiety followed by an unconscious somatic and emotional retreat into a cocoon of not living 'in her external world' through thinking, talking, walking or eating.

'Gathering the transference' to the therapist is an important aspect of psychoanalytic psychotherapy (Meltzer, 1967) and my task was to consider the evolving nature of Yufang's relationship with me as a reiteration of her internal conflicts. In the initial sessions I felt I was to be present to simply experience and contain within myself a flow of Yufang's undifferentiated feelings and sensations. By the fifth week there was a splitting process developing in her transference relationship with me. On the one hand, she was able to dream, remember the dream and share two words of it, which suggests a developing trust in me and a growing faith in the emotionally containing, thinking process which therapy provided. Her growing dependence upon me aroused a protective, distrustful part of her opposed to talking with me, so she bit her lip that had been trying to talk with me.

There is an oscillation between different physical/emotional responses: Yufang cries, coughs, lets mucous run from her nose as though trying to let out some noxious substances and experiences. In these situations she is aware of something 'not good', 'not pleasant' needing to erupt from her body. States of boredom, going blank or yawning reflect massive denial and when she giggles it seems there is an increase in the force within her against sharing her experiences and thinking about them with me (Rosenfeld, 1987a).

Attacks on her actual skin on her fingers, the biting of her lips and then the somatization of pain and aggression to her legs which felt pain, and later her heart and chest during the Christmas break, suggest that her rage goes underground to the internalized objects of her internal world and thus protects the external figures, her parents and me, from her rage (Symington, 2002). But the question remains, what developmental level is being experienced by Yufang? I had the distinct impression that we were experiencing together her very earliest infantile anxieties of being attached to the protective, nurturing mother and feeling that she was falling into an abyss when separating. By the fifth week, Yufang seemed to be losing her balance so that I had to prevent her from falling. Her reluctance to leave the session suggested to me that she now had become attached to the 'thinking space' with me. Being left by me at the end of the session and between the sessions left her feeling 'dropped by me'. The falling is a dramatization of how the child in her feels dropped. If I do not hold her in my mind all the time she falls down again and again, can't walk and lets the bits of her mind fall apart. If Yufang depends on me and I leave her, the time feels so limitless, like that of a newborn not feeling certain mother will return and this affects both Yufang's body and her mind.

I talked directly with Yufang about feeling I dropped her. Simultaneously I wondered to myself if her leg pains were linked with her anger with me for walking away from her. Perhaps her anger became unconsciously diverted towards the internal object: she attacked my legs walking away from her and identified with me and my damaged legs. By the sixth week Yufang was hanging onto my arm, not wanting to separate at all lest in our separation she would begin to psychologically and physically fragment and fall apart entirely.

An eighth-week session

It is the last session before the Christmas holidays. Yufang does not speak. She yawns but seems to be in a manic excited state. After she has given me a wrapped tin of cherry tea, I thank her and later I again discuss my Christmas break, which will last for ten days. Immediately, Yufang seems to see something dancing before her eyes. She begins to giggle. I feel that she is in a dizzy, confused state which minimizes the impact of what I am saying. Later she turns to me and three or four times makes some very ugly smiling-monster faces and then laughs. I suggest, 'I am to feel scared by a "bad cruel monster,"' as I witness her shockingly frightening and grotesque faces. When I take out the family dolls and describe, 'You will be going home for a few hours on Christmas day,' Yufang says, 'My mother is a very, very good cook,' adding, 'I like my mother's food.' I tell Yufang, 'Now there is a good, loving mother who gives you love and good food.' When I put the dolls back into their container, for the first time she comments. 'The dolls are being flattened!' Later in the day, the doctors are called to investigate Yufang's severe chest pains, discovering them to be without a physical basis. When the doctors examine her, she becomes sexually excited and temporarily manic. I wonder if Yufang is again dramatically feeling, in her body, her emotional experiences of 'being flattened' by my departure, my putting her away. The sexual excitement created by the doctors' touch then pulls her from a flattened 'low state' into a manic state.

Comments on the eighth-week session

I described to Yufang how there was a sense of happy, dancing figures cruelly looking down at the 'child-Yufang' who was feeling the separation from me. Initially it seemed Yufang was hallucinating cruel faces. She identified with these cruel figures, imitating their faces, while I was to be the terrified child facing monstrous faces. In contrast to this, there existed a very good mother who made good meals and stayed with 'the little girl Yufang', looking after her, not going away at Christmas time like me. I thought Yufang was showing off this 'good providing mother' to foster jealousy in me, but I was relieved that now she had a sense of something good. Experiences were no longer 'all bad'. When we parted for the Christmas break I realized Yufang had given me a gift to show her appreciation, but I recalled feeling flat inside as we were nearing the end of the session. I interpreted my leaving as squashing her, making her feel the life was being squashed out of her... as she had shown by her squashing the dolls back into the box. The pain in Yufang's chest/heart suggested once again that the therapist inside is being attacked for being uncaring and leaving her.

A ninth-week session

When I return from the Christmas break, Yufang cries profusely and then feels her stomach. I respond, 'I feel your tears.' She replies, 'Not crying.' Then she is silent. I suggest, 'You are crying but you do not want to be close to the pain.' After a long pause Yufang queries, 'What is the difference between belief and trust?' She then cries more profusely. I wonder aloud, 'Can you trust me enough to tell me what you are feeling?' Her lip trembles with incredible sadness and tears flow down her cheeks. I say, 'You may have been very sad while I was away.' She mumbles some inaudible words. I say, 'You are relieved that I have come back. You weren't sure I would.' After a long while Yufang says, with a hint of pleasure, 'My brother is coming in the spring.' Being projected into me is a feeling of being unimportant, a feeling that perhaps Yufang has had when I left her. Simultaneously I realize that

Yufang is beginning to hold onto some hope of having good experiences in the future and having me return was in itself a good experience for her.

An 18th-week session

When finally a vacancy on the inpatient psychiatric unit became available, Yufang's medical condition had improved so much that Yufang, her parents and the consultant psychiatrist decided that she was well enough to be cared for at home. The decision was based partly on the fact that the consultant psychiatrist felt that Yufang was making good use of six times per week psychotherapy and agreed for her to have outpatient psychotherapy three times per week and begin two cello lessons per week in order to put some structure into her days.

Yufang missed the first outpatient appointment, because her mother was unable to bring her. On the second appointment she arrives wearing a new white long sleeved blouse, looking like an elegant woman in *Vogue* magazine. She apologizes for missing the first appointment and says that since she couldn't come she decided to write for the first time and put some thoughts in a notebook. During the four days we have not met she has written haiku-style poem which she reads dramatically following each word with a pause:

> Night star, moon wind
> noise, light, shine, whisper
> sound, a hint, a code.
> Be fragrant, silent
> warmth, asleep
> The moment of silence
> hanging in the air.

She has also drawn a cartoon-style picture of her beloved grandmother who is in China. On the next page is an airplane which she says symbolizes a film she has seen on the day of her missed session. At my request she describes the film, saying:

> A plane was searching for a man who fell near Mt. McKinley. Someone was calling out from the mountain, 'Naomi, Naomi'. The man died near the foot of the mountain.

Yufang then reads out the words on the last page of her notebook:

> If I had a scoop of melon,
> the world will be all right.
> If all the houses are upset

but tree won't move other place.
Space is all round, round and round.
I can hear the voice from another space.
I have to do something, my mind go fast.
I broke the window.
That is mad but not mad.

There is an empty white space on the sheet beside the poem and Yufang tells me it is 'a glass window'. She says, 'I wanted to break through the glass window and throw myself out of the window. I wanted to do that when I was ill.'

Comments on 18th-week session

The move from inpatient to outpatient psychotherapy was an important transition and it was accompanied by Yufang missing the first session. What is impressive is that Yufang could be an active participant in gathering together and trying to make sense of the multitude of emotions racing through her mind. I strove for simplicity in the session because too many feelings were threatening to deluge her. Gradually I let her know:

> You have missed the session which is very unusual for you. You felt the silence of the missed session, felt very lost. When we didn't meet you began trying to find some ways of taking care of yourself. You found a notebook, writing down your thoughts and your dream.

I also described, 'How terrible it felt inside when you risked letting those feelings get too big and take you over.'

I was aware of, but did not comment on the fact, that today she had slipped into the identity of 'a fashionable, beautiful mother' in her silk blouse in an attempt to 'hold herself together' and she was continuing to do so. At this point, what was important was that she was making attempts to contain her emotions in whatever ways she could through giving them symbolic expression rather than to deny them or somatize them. This is a very significant step forward for such Yufang who had been such a severely ill, near-death young person.

A session in the 22nd week

Yufang arrives with a little straw nest holding three tiny toy bluebirds. Some feathers are scattered around the nest. She tells me this dream:

> Military officers from two countries were hiding behind trees. It was midnight, the men were shooting at me. I was a boy. I was standing there questioning, 'What was the best way to die?' I thought to myself, 'Fast

firing guns are better than dying slowly.' There were many children with families in the dream.

When I asked Yufang for associations to the dream she replied, 'In primary school there were three children who were angry with me and I didn't know why ... When I was in China I was angry with my mother.'

Comments on the 22nd-week session

In this session Yufang seemed to be expressing her conscious wish to preserve the babies of the mother represented by the three birds in the nest. I sensed that there was a hint of compassion, suggesting the development of a good, loving, sensitive aspect of herself – necessary for reparation of damaged internal figures. However, Yufang also seemed to be aware that there was a destructive force inside her from which 'these families with children' required protection. Yufang describes herself as feeling anger towards 'the mother'. In her dream there is shooting, representing on some level her own 'shooting feelings'. A boy is being shot. A boomerang effect of her own aggression occurs in the form of violent, punitive, persecutory guilt represented by the soldiers shooting her. She seems rather fascinated by the killing, asking, 'Which is better, slow or fast killing?'

Yufang not only writes and draws to symbolize her feelings when awake, she is also dreaming and bringing her dreams to symbolize her inner conflicts and to gain understanding. An inner space for dreaming and giving words to feelings is emerging. I begin to contemplate that what contributed significantly to Yufang's regression and 'near-death' was Yufang's inner conflicts, including her difficulty in acknowledging hostile feelings, augmented by the weight of the external trauma which included massive losses through separation from her country, grandmother, brother and first boyfriend.

Yufang's three times weekly psychotherapy continued for three years until sadly it was stopped by her parents. They felt that there was no reason for her to continue therapy when ostensibly she was so much better. I felt she needed more time in therapy to consolidate her inner psychological development, but the parents did not agree. Yufang felt she had no choice but to go along with her parents' decision.

Yufang had developed more capacity to stay with a feeling, lend thought to it and make decisions accordingly. Projecting feelings into others had diminished considerably and I felt she was more able to intro-jectively identify with 'the good internal mother' rather than just slip into my shoes in an imitative fashion. Yufang was very successful in her new cello studies at an excellent music academy and felt pleasure in describing to me how she loved her music and was playing with more feeling than ever before. With some shyness, but with much enjoyment, she described her pleasure in socializing with both British and Chinese friends. I still felt

Yufang had a very fragile state without sufficient emotional capacity to understand and hold her extremely passionate feelings. I heard later that she successfully graduated from the musical academy and had regained her capacity to remember and to think more about her emotional conflicts.

Chapter 8

Understanding the imprisoned self

A different kind of taming

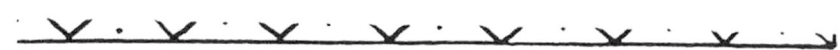

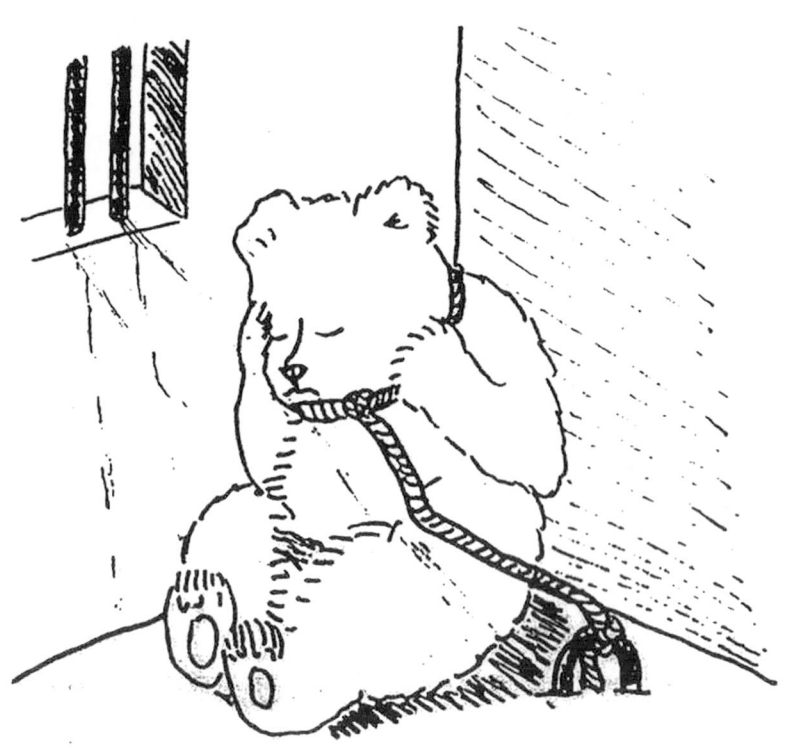

Figure 8.1 A bear in a prison cell

DOI: 10.4324/9781003044970-9

Introduction

'She hates me,' I told the team when describing my psychotherapy session with 13-year-old Pakistani girl, Amal. Suffering from anorexia nervosa, Amal had just had her fourth psychotherapy session in an inpatient setting. However, I was too awkward to mention that I felt nothing I could say or do seemed to feel any good to her. I felt like 'poison food' to Amal, an unwanted intruder into her life.

At times outside her session time, as I walk past her in the corridor and greet her, Amal walks by me, her eyes turned downward. She does not smile at me, does not look at me: her whole body posture remains unchanging, as though I do not exist. I have not spoken. 'Why do I deserve this?' I ask myself. 'I have hardly spoken to her, she does not know me.' Once again I feel 'no good', thrown away like some long ago discarded, useless piece of clothing. I am avoided in the same way that Amal avoids food.

Actually, I often find myself reflecting on this sort of situation I experience as a psychotherapist. Why do I work with people having such severe eating disorders? What is the attraction of embarking on a job in an Eating Disorders Unit having 20 young people aged nine to 18? For what reasons do I engage in psychotherapy with young people who frequently 'barricade themselves', shutting themselves off from their parents, their friends, the nurses, doctors and psychotherapists, and from themselves?

Initially in my encounters with anorectic young people, the vulnerable self remains unconscious and often imprisoned in the most dramatic ways. Figure 8.1 shows an example, in a picture drawn by another anorectic girl in psychotherapy with me.

Returning now to Amal: she had initially stopped eating and drinking completely. This had been preceded by her using 'not-thinking': moving into not knowing her feelings, a kind of freezing of access both to her conscious and unconscious self-awareness. For example,

- Amal had difficulty in sleeping, but had no access to her dreams.
- She was lonely, but had no access to words for her emotions.
- Her body was cold and tired, but she seemed to have no sensation of heat, cold or tiredness.

During her fifth session I continued to try to talk with Amal. I did not do this so much by asking her questions, for I understood that questions did indeed make me a demandingly curious and intrusive figure. Rather I merely continued to reflect upon how she was being, what it must be like for her in my presence. Apart from a few irritated and cold comments made to correct me, Amal stood looking out the window with her back firmly to me, her face invisible. Later she curled up into a foetal position with her head tucked into her body as if guarding against access to her heart.

After this session I found myself once again pondering over the questions:

- Why have I chosen to work in a situation where initially I am so constantly rejected?
- Why have I chosen to sit out in the cold, in the silence, while my thoughts are given voice, only to fall flat to the ground?

I feel that I cannot go any further with Amal until I understand my own countertransference experiences and my decision to work with her and those specific anorectic young people who, apart from their initial compliant entry into the consulting room, for a period of time, either covertly or overtly completely reject me, and what I represent.

Eating disorder specialists often focus on ways of helping young people become motivated to start eating again; there is discussion about calories, methods of achieving weight gain, comorbidity, perfectionism, transcultural issues, genetic predisposition, obsessionality, cognitive behaviour therapy and textbook family therapy. All of these issues may be important; however, they generally do not address the young person's central issue regarding her specific relationship with her therapist or her *Core Self.* Nor do many professionals address the issue of why any of us would want to work with young people like Amal, starving themselves to death, self-harming through scratching, and apparently rejecting psychotherapy and the therapist as a person.

Twenty years ago it was fascinating to learn about all the different aspects of anorexia nervosa; but now I have become bored and too familiar with the sameness of 'the international unhealthy club' of anorexia nervosa, in which all the members, regardless of their culture, colour or creed, sexual identity or gender, appear united in performing similar patterns of starving, calorie counting, exercising, hating their bodies, which are felt to be both ugly and fat, hating themselves. I ask myself:

What is the appeal for me of being exposed to this day in and day out? Nothing! There must be something far more important here to me personally than simply having a useful salaried job as a psychoanalytic individual and family psychotherapist.

So again I ask myself: 'What is it? Why expose myself to so much lack of love for the self and for me?' At times, if you are working with eating disordered young people, you probably find yourselves asking the same question. Probably for each of us there will probably be different answers, all of them potentially important. I shall fumble through my thoughts and feelings to try to answer the question subjectively: 'Why have I chosen to work with so much rejection of all that is me?'

As I allow my thoughts to wander, I recall Rilke's (1981, p. 65) unpublished poem:

Oh misery, my mother tears me down.
Stone upon stone I'd laid, towards a Self
And stood like a small house, with day's expanse around it,
Now comes my mother, comes and tears me down.
She tears me down by coming and looking,
That someone builds she does not see.
Right through my wall of stones she walks for me.
Oh misery, my mother tears me down...

I also think of Emily Dickenson's poem that I chanted as a budding adolescent:

I am Nobody. Who are You?
Are you – Nobody – Too?
Then there's a pair of us.
Don't tell! They'd banish us – you know!
How dreary to be Somebody
How public – like a Frog –
To tell one's name – the livelong day
To an admiring Bog.
(Dickinson, 1861, p. 43)

Despite my having had a very close group of school friends, there must have been some attack on my internal mother and my internal siblings to identify with feeling 'I am nobody' rather than feeling I am 'somebody'.

In my cogitations about why I am willing to work in an environment of rejection, I review one of my naturalistic observations of infants and children at home with their mothers and fathers.

I remember one-month-old Jane, rapturous as she looks into her mother's eyes and feels the beauty of being received into her gaze. Her mother is delighted to have given birth to a healthy baby so responsive to her love.

As the weeks pass, I see Jane crying as her mother leaves the room. When she hears the sound of her mother's footsteps walking down the corridor, Jane stops crying.

When, at eight months, Jane begins to crawl, she follows her mother from the sitting room into the adjoining kitchen. Jane gazes intently at her mother talking to father, making tea and then sitting at the table to assist her brother, Jeremy, with a puzzle.

When mother is not carefully watching her children, Jane gets hit by her 18-month-old brother Jeremy. But Jane no longer cries when this occurs. Instead she stops breathing, remains motionless and hiccups.

Mother finds it difficult to give Jane what she needs because she is worried about inciting Jeremy's jealousy. Jane is often left alone while mother reads stories and plays with Jeremy.

One day Jane pours her cereal on top of her head and leaves the table. Gradually she stops following her mother around, because she finds that mother is always playing with Jeremy. Instead Jane turns to her blue blanket, containing all the lovely smells of herself and mother being together. Often left alone, still aged under 15 months, Jane 'reads' her own storybooks.

As time progresses, Jane begins to develop a different relationship with her mother. At 15 months she is perfectly capable of playing on her own. She is described as a 'good baby' who rarely cries. By 17 months Jane has developed a wide range of words and an interest in little picture books and some toys. By the time she is two, Jane is able to speak in complete sentences.

Jane's intellect goes on developing in a most impressive way. She is top in her primary school classes. In her mind she has to be top in the class or she has failed. She has to do each sentence in her homework perfectly, with perfect spelling or she has failed once again. There is an obsessional way in which her school project on Great Britain's terrain has to be redone again and again until it looks both beautiful and perfect. As if in compensation for feeling rejected and unprotected by mother, Jane is extremely hardworking, continually needing to achieve recognition and 'A stars'. Through her 'A stars' she hopes to win her parents' love and the acclaim of her teachers representing them.

As time went on I felt that Jane had split off a part of her ego, separating her vulnerable, emotional self from her intellectual achieving self. Part of her was still the ten-month-old baby. This self was fiercely protected by an omnipotent, pseudo-mature protective structure.

This observation of baby Jane's childhood comes to mind when 13-year-old Amal says, 'I would like to be five years old again because I would be able to play with my small furry toys.' She later describes,

> I've been being 'grown up' for too many years! I was very good when I was little. Then no one noticed how I was feeling. Now I am going to remain anorectic: then my mother can feed me and look after me forever!

Before being hospitalized for her anorexia, Amal wouldn't separate from her mother; her mother had to stay with her every meal and always keep a careful eye on her. Feeling jealous, Amal hit her older 14-year-old sister, Rukkiya, when she attempted to talk to their mother.

Amal says that she has no space in the family. She often goes into her room and closes the door: then she has physical space, but that does not mean she has space in the family. Her mother said that when Amal was little she tried to cuddle Amal, but Amal rejected her. Amal says that sometimes her mother comes into her room to try to talk with her or encourage her to come downstairs to be with the family, but she rejects her mother. She does not feel she has a space in the family because it is too chaotic. Amal is feeling lonely but she has created an omnipotent, 'I can take care of myself' self which is threatened by, and fends off, every affectionate or understanding gesture made by her mother or me.

However, in a surprisingly cooperative moment, Amal draws a picture of a 22-year-old girl with a dog curled up beside her.

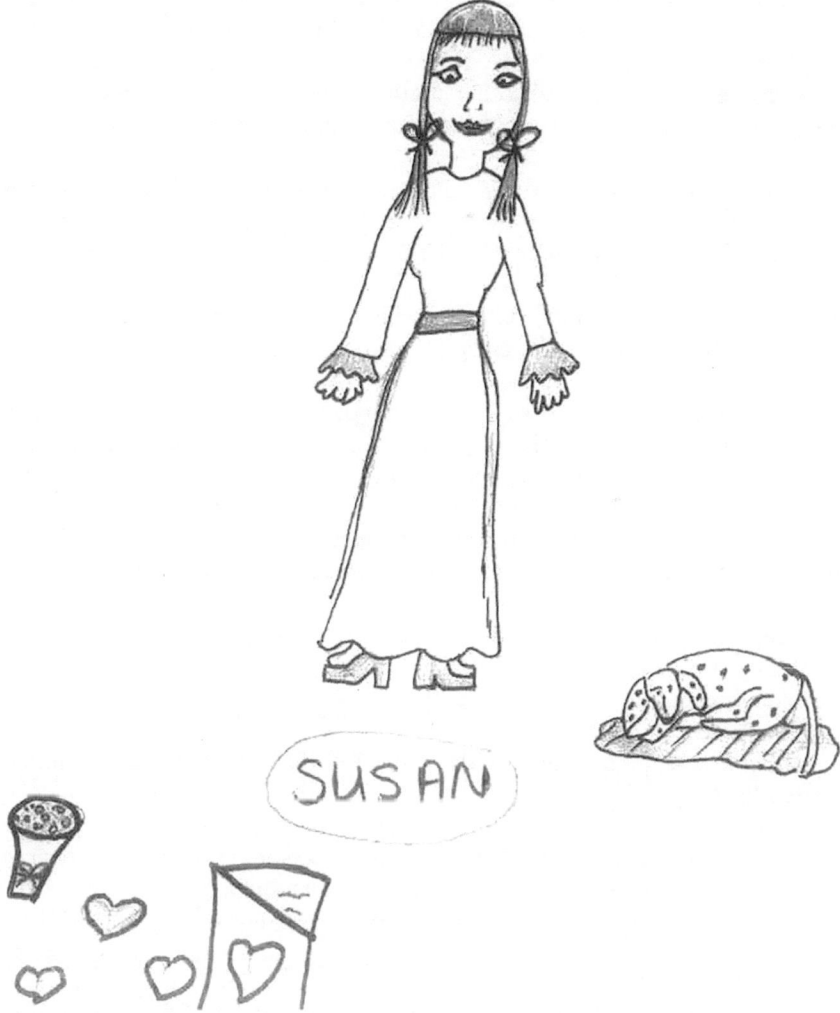

Figure 8.2 A girl with a curled up dog

When I look at the picture, I think of Amal's teacher's remark: 'Either she is 18 or she is five … there is no maturity enabling her to be her own age, 13.'

Primitive omnipotence

Now I would like to consider Amal's use of primitive omnipotence. There is an infantile part of Amal's personality, which feels very thin-skinned and it embodies Amal's terrorized, fearing, loving, hating and angry emotions. The eyes of the 22-year-old look worried. Her feelings are excessive and frightening in their intensity now because they are infantile emotions which were never experienced sufficiently consciously or expressed openly, when Amal was a baby. Amal, like the baby Jane described in the earlier case study, was described as 'a quiet, good baby'. Now when Amal lets out her feelings they are overwhelming to her and to her mother. She screams out, cries, hits her mother. She speaks to me sharply but with a hint of plaintiveness, saying,

> You don't understand me, how could you understand me! You just pretend you know me. You don't know who I really am! I don't like you, I don't like being here. I don't like home. I don't like who I am. I don't like being me!

The curled up dog and Amal curled up behind the couch contain fears of disintegration, falling to pieces, dissolving into a state of nothingness with no thing existing, no body, no self. The 22-year-old girl seems to represent a Self repeatedly using omnipotence and a series of primitive protective mechanisms. Esther Bick (1968), describes how this series of primitive protective mechanisms are used in early infancy to maintain some cohesion of the Self. The primitive protective mechanisms are brought into play when there is a break in a connection with mother, or in the absence of an emotionally empathic, physically holding, loving and understanding mother. These primitive protective mechanisms include:

- Denial.
- Bodily constriction and erotization.
- Omniscience.
- Omnipotence.
- Adherence to pathological parts of the Self dictating Self-starvation and Self-harm.

In a moment of crisis or conflict, the child or person of any age can turn to an inner or outer emotionally receptive or understanding mother or to any one of these primitive protective mechanisms. Over-use of any one of these protective mechanisms involves not turning to an understanding mother or the unavailability of a mother who would recognize and tolerate psychic pain, love and longing as well as hate and rage. For example, the child can turn to the harsh superego and over-use of the intellectual functions, self-harm or anorexia as part of a rescue operation when the Self fears disintegration. Also the child may fear losing mother's love or fear destroying mother's emotional stability if she shows hostility towards her.

Self-harm as part of the total transference

I shall now look at Amal's scratching and my thoughts about self-harm in anorectic young people. Self-harm may well have been part of a young person's history prior to her embarking upon psychotherapy. Once therapy has commenced, it is essential that the psychotherapist takes the scratching, cutting and overdosing into the total transference to the therapist. By this I mean that the whole of the child's emotional response to the inpatient environment (the setting, institutional procedures, the range of staff functions) needs to be understood as part of the total transference relationship to the therapist. When Amal speaks of being 'caged in' and 'locked up' I assume that she is talking about being trapped not only by anorectic ideas, her parents' decision to admit her to an inpatient unit, and the nurses caring for her, but also by her becoming claustrophobic during this voyage involving interacting with me in a required individual psychotherapy.

In my experience a greater risk of self-harm emerges once the young person begins to be more aware of the usefulness of the therapist and her increasingly vulnerable dependence on the therapist's understanding as a source of relief and understanding. At this point in therapy the young person has begun to let go of some of the primitive omnipotence involving denial of feelings and the obsessive control involved in being anorectic, exercising and starving herself. As a result, self-harm can increase if the young person feels overwhelmed by the wave of liberated infantile feelings particularly in relation to separation from the therapist or the therapist's misattunement. It is for this reason it is important before the therapist's holiday to find and discuss traces of the young person's panic or pain regarding the therapist's absence. Also it is important for the therapist to notice ruptures in the therapeutic relationship and find ways with the young person to mend them.

I have noticed that therapists' responses to self-harm often involve too great a need to be liked by the patient, a difficulty in tolerating the experience of being a bad persecutory figure, and a tendency to 'split the transference' of the young person so that the therapist receives the loving transference and talks about 'the bad outside world' as seen by the patient her relationships with parents, friends, teachers, nursing staff. The failure to take the young person's rage, hostility and sense of abandonment into the total transference to the therapist (Meltzer, 1967, p. 20; Joseph, 1985) can lead to terrible acting out by the child's vulnerable, infantile part in relation to both the inpatient staff and the parents. It can also promote the young person's scratching, cutting and overdosing.

There are various factors that tend to seduce the therapist into gathering the young person's positive, loving transference while allowing her negative transference to be split off and directed to auxiliary staff, parents, teachers, the peers:

- The therapist falsely assumes that the patient is securely attached to the therapist and simultaneously the therapist's need to feel loved by the patient prevents the therapist from acknowledging the patient's hostility.

- The ambivalently attached patient does not trust the therapist to receive her hostility without rejecting her. The patient then denies her hostility to the therapist, appears to be getting along with the therapist, while attacking the therapist internally. As a result the patient has an internalized revengeful therapist who appears, for example, in nightmares of being attacked by the psychotherapist. Figure 8.3 is an illustration of such a nightmare: a witch-therapist with biting teeth and scratching nails.

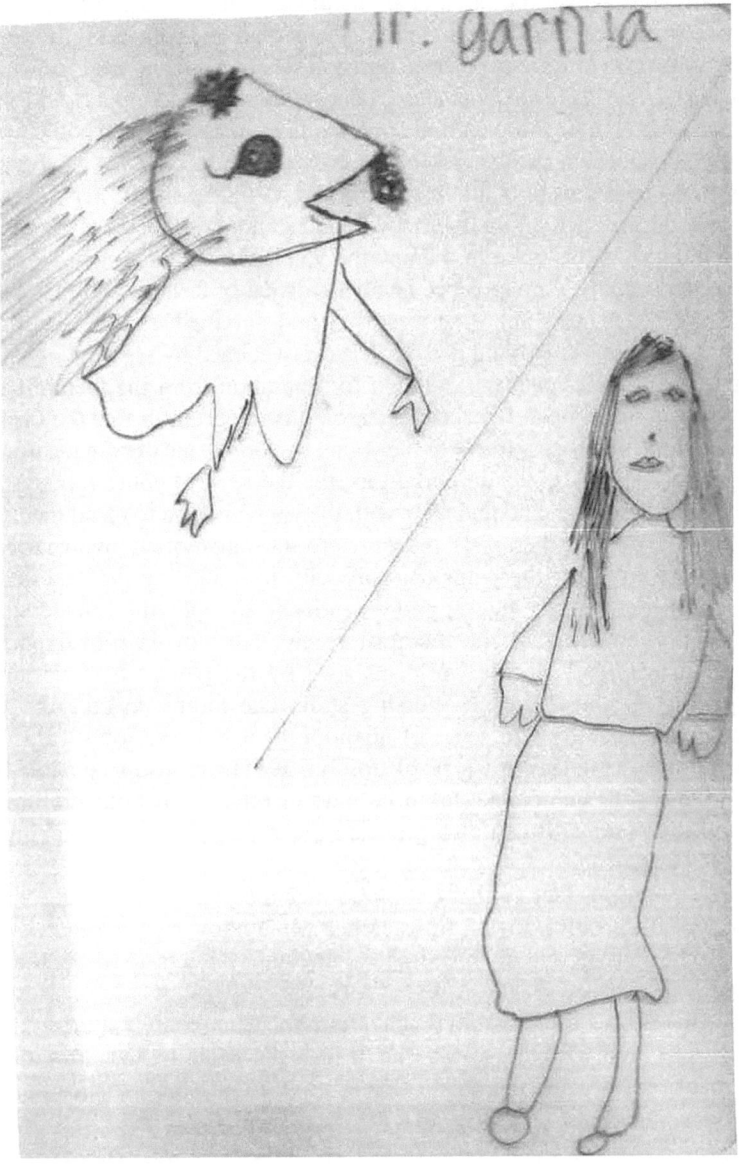

Figure 8.3 'Witch-therapist'

The young person drawing this picture is denying her hostility to the external mother represented by the therapist. (At one point six of the eight anorectic young people in our therapy group were terrified by the thought of attacks by spiders filled with their projections of hostility.) As well as unconscious hostility, one girl consciously hid her cutting, saying, 'I wanted you to think well of me. I was afraid of what you would think if I told you.'

- The anxiously attached patient seems overly possessive. The therapist has not sufficiently integrated her own experiences of rejection and her own latent destructiveness in the face of it. Thus she is blinded to the patient's lack of a good internal therapist and resulting sense of helplessness, her sense of total despair at being left without any good object internally to give her sense of security and her panic as well as hostility and rage towards the abandoning therapist.

- An avoidant attachment to the therapist can present even more difficulties for the therapist to tolerate: for the isolated, pseudo-competent, intellectualizing young person's heart seems hard and unreceptive to the therapist. It is then, only by looking at the young person's unconscious communication, in the themes of the stories and in the young person's dreams and drawings that the young person's sense of being 'dropped' by the therapist is visible.

Some dreams predicting and describing current reactions to feeling dropped by the therapist include:

- Night after night, I dreamt I was falling down the stairs.
- I dreamt I was in a hotel and couldn't find my way around.
- I dreamt I went to the train station, but as I arrived I discovered my train was departing.
- I dreamt that all the girls and staff liked Serena's cheerfulness, but no one liked me.

Often, after two to four months of a psychotherapy which is going reasonably well, several phenomena occur virtually simultaneously: the young person begins to have more trust in the therapist's capacity to be useful to her and the psychotherapist takes a holiday. This is at a time when the therapist must take particular care in preparing the young person for separation and understand the young person's sense that when *therapist and young person are not joined together, the therapist will be experienced* as a rejecting mother, evoking all the eating disordered young person's infantile experiences of rejecting figures from the past. It is essential for the therapist to understand carefully his or her own feelings and countertransference responses connected with leaving the young person between sessions, or experiencing lapses in empathy during the session, or taking a holiday. The young person's unconscious self also feels abandoned *by the therapist* even when it is the young person who has missed a regular psychotherapy session.

Often the therapy is progressing without additional self-harm, apart from starvation, until the first break in therapy schedule, or the therapist's first internal crisis created by her own lack of empathy for the young person. Lack of empathy and understanding as well as separation from the therapist can mean that the young person feels torn away, thrown away by the therapist's lack of understanding, or emotional or physical absence. Rage about unmet needs, but also a possessive rage and panic about separation, are often some of the fundamental issues which are evaded, but need addressing in working psychotherapeutically with an eating disordered young person.

Understanding one's countertransference

Often I find myself or a supervisee saying, 'I have a difficult patient who needs to be understood.' Nowadays, I immediately spot a problem when I say this. Let me give you an example:

Fourteen-year-old anorectic Lorna is adhesively clinging in an anxious attachment to me. She is very possessive towards me and I discover through her dream about an Old English sheepdog in a garden that she has found my private home address and is regularly visiting my dog through the fence in the garden when I am away at work. Discovering her intrusiveness and possessiveness of me feels so overwhelming that unfortunately I become sleepy and move into a kind of non-thinking in a session with her. On the following evening she took an overdose of paracetamol and was required to have her stomach contents pumped out.

It was not simply that I had a difficult patient but rather that I had difficulty in the countertransference: I had not been able to become conscious of, understand or bear, Lorna's possessive, clinging relationship towards me.

In exploring the overdose and what needed to change for it not to happen again, I discovered that I was indeed the only person upon whom Lorna could depend. She had been having a sexual relationship with her alcoholic mother's boyfriend. Her betrayal of her alcoholic mother, who did not perceive the ongoing sexual abuse, led Lorna to fear rejection by everyone in her life. She was also afraid of what would happen if she revealed the sexual relationship with her mother's boyfriend. But as a young trainee psychotherapist, I was afraid... afraid to accept Lorna's total dependence on me, in the absence of a supportive family outside the therapy.

Lorna's overdose made me aware that the problem is often not simply a 'difficult patient', but the countertransference difficulty in being open to the truth of the burden of the cruel, painful, vulnerable, dependent feelings of Lorna and Amal and all those other young people with whom I work in therapy. I now acknowledge that both the psychotherapist's and anorectic young person's vulnerable emotional self may be 'imprisoned' in various ways.

It is not only intellectual knowledge about anorexia nervosa that is needed but also emotional space for the psychotherapist to understand what the young person is stirring up in the depths of her own psyche.

These countertransference conflicts which need to be understood in relation to questions such as:

- Why is the patient running away at just the time of her session?
- Why is the patient taking an overdose just that time?
- How does she feel about leaving me and the inpatient unit with no adequate external support when she leaves?
- Why does she starve, scratch, cut, overdose more on the weekends when I and her keyworkers are not around?

In a busy schedule, one might choose to read books on anorexia and relax by reading novels rather than look at one's countertransference conflicts that are the heart of the matter of the young person's and therapist's psychological development together. In particular if the therapist has many people in psychotherapy, the risk is that inadequate time is given to examine the young person's deep transference to the therapist, and the therapist's response and her difficulties in maintaining an open, empathic, and understanding connection to the young person. Racker's (1974) book *Transference and Countertransference*, Rosenfeld's (1987a) book *Impasse and Interpretation* and one's own self-analysis in which one freely associates to that which the young person has brought during the session are particularly important aides to repairing the damaged connection between psychotherapist and young person.

One of the chief problems in working with Amal is that the 22-year-old, strong backed, rejecting girl speaks through body language, silence and with very few words to me. The 'curled up puppy' part of her is barely, if at all, consciously available to her. Amal's 'curled up puppy' part does not speak directly but rather through acting out conflictual issues with me. I find that I have been so overwhelmed by 'the rejecting 22-year-old Amal' that it has been difficult for me to even notice the positive, clinging feelings of 'the curled up puppy', Amal. That is why supervision is so helpful.

In our multidisciplinary team's weekly review meeting, the head-teacher pointed at the 'curled up infantile' part of Amal in the drawing and said to me, 'You say she hates you, but there is more to it than that.' The teacher had noted that several times Amal stood to the side of the staff dining table, carefully watching me eating and talking to colleagues. This timely interjection alerted me to the interested, curious, dependent, loving feelings of 'the curled up puppy' Amal: her vulnerable, infantile self that is imprisoned behind the rejecting 22-year-old 'hard back to me' Amal.

After the sixth session I had to rearrange a session. Amal acted as though she hadn't heard; however, in response to this news, when I greeted her for the subsequent session she said she had some Spanish homework to do: that she had to do it and would like to miss the session to do it. When I suggested that we meet to talk about her dilemma, rather than miss the session, Amal was furious with me. I did not immediately understand Amal's unconscious projection of her feeling that I had broken up the rhythm of our sessions together and abandoned her on the actual day of her session. She gave me a 'hard rejection' in identification with my abandoning therapist self. I missed this because I could only see the 'hard reject-ing' Amal. 'Make-up' sessions on a different day and at a different time, no matter how good they are, can never be the same as the regular session within the regular rhythm of the week. The more verbal young people repeatedly tell me this.

Understanding the total transference of the young person means giving meaning to denied feelings of 'the imprisoned self' that appear in dreams and acting out, or through unconscious sentiments expressed in stories of external events. That is why it is so important to look at the unconscious non-verbalized communication of the 'imprisoned self' which speaks via tone of voice, body posture, dreams, and acting out, often in identification with the aggressor. I have found it very useful to see the so-called 'resistance' of the young person as her protective armour: protecting the her from the agony of the dependent infantile self in the transference. Such protection may have been needed earlier in life and now it has become established as an aspect of her personality which impedes intimacy in relationships.

'To love is to become a beggar' says former anorectic Kathryn Harrison in a poem regarding her mother, 'Mother's Day Card' (2003), which she read on the radio:

> I still dream of you …
> Even in sleep I'm paralyzed by desire …
> How can I hold you? How can I keep you?
> I wake exhausted from the excitement of your presence.
> Long ago love made me a beggar, grateful for a glimpse of the hem of your dress brushing past. I have missed you all my life!

A child who feels love immediately suffers the agony of missing. The anorectic young person, while deep down longing to be loved, has generally had an ambivalent relationship with her mother and father. Opening a dialogue with both Amal's 'protective functioning 22-year-old armour' and her 'imprisoned infantile self' is essential at some point, but we must remember that underneath the anorexia nervosa is the cruel, perfectionist self, demanding that not only the young person but also the therapist get it absolutely right.

I am not sure that the imprisoned self is mature enough to understand or even use words, because much infantile experience is still unsymbolized and stored in the brain's non-declarative part. A two-month-old baby I saw a few days ago cried when mother took away the breast. Mother was distracted and did not notice how enraged the baby was. When, belatedly, the mother returned her nipple to her screaming baby, the baby turned her head away terrified, as though the nipple was a sword intruding into her. She screamed and for a long time could not be comforted. This baby does not yet understand words: all her communications are at the behavioural, sensori-motor and sensori-affective levels and will be stored in the brain's non-declarative part.

Likewise I expect that although I will try to find suitable words or images for the experience of 'the imprisoned self', the 'hard, armoured' Amal will hardly comprehend what I am talking about. Hence it is essential to be aware of all her nonverbal communications and how I attune to them through my verbal and nonverbal responses to her tone of voice, gesture, play, touch, eye contact. The 'imprisoned infantile self' is almost as foreign to her as it is to me. She insists there is nothing inside. Yet I know the infantile self has its 'foreign language' with messages that seem unintelligible and foreign to both Amal and me. I cannot see the infantile transference and she certainly is not conscious of any dependence on me that involves feeling unsettled about having the rhythm of our sessions changed. We will have to comprehend the 'foreign language' and unravel its meaning together. Also I have homework to do after the session so that I understand and more effectively communicate what I feel in the countertransference. I felt harshly rejected by Amal's decision to skip me for her Spanish homework, but I didn't not know how to speak about it.

She grips my heart without words. Present in the imprisoned self is a sense not only of being rejected by a therapist leaving her, but also of a distracted therapist thinking selfishly about what she wants to do… such as attending a meeting or conference or having a holiday. This is not just a sense of being rejected but rather because the therapist is simply 'a stupid therapist' (Alvarez, 2012) who does not understand what is going on in the 'imprisoned self'.

As the therapy deepens there often arises, in relation to the therapist from the imprisoned self, years of denied hurt and hostility to the parents and siblings.

For example, in response to the first rearranged session, Amal had scratched her wrists slightly and had refused to eat over the weekend. It is convenient for me to think to myself, 'Well, it had nothing to do with me. I wasn't present during the interaction between her and the staff or her and her parents.' But to look at behaviour in an inpatient unit as simply belonging elsewhere denudes me of responsibility of being in the total transference that is represented also by the institution and parents. I certainly feel that Amal also has some responsibility; however, she does not know the emotions of 'the imprisoned self'; they are foreign to her because they have been projected or imprisoned for a very long time. They come alive in the infantile transference to me where they can be acknowledged, understood and integrated within her personality in order that she can grow up – so she won't forever have to be just a five or a 22-year-old.

Until I can establish a better rapport with '22-year-old Amal', who is actually 13, I am going to have a hard time talking to her 'infantile imprisoned self'. All I can do is muse aloud … or tell stories with or without the stuffed animals and puppets that I have brought, just in case, into the session with me. I tell stories about others, not her, through talking to the puppets.

Sometimes the stories are about animals because they are less threatening as examples than humans, which feel too close to Amal for comfort.

Here is one story I told:

> You know, Amal, I had a dog once. The dog seemed to accept whatever I did and whatever happened. It was so strange. I had to teach my dog to bark. The dog and I became very friendly with one another. Then I went on a holiday and had someone else look after my dog. My dog wouldn't eat. Instead she just chewed up my shoe, something which she had never done before. It was a puzzle. That left me always wondering why that had occurred. I didn't realize that my absence would have such an effect on my dog.

At this stage in the therapy, I feel I may have to sit silently with some of my countertransference experiences. However, through the dog story I gave a space for us to acknowledge what I hadn't really understood – that, although Amal was overtly rejecting, I was important to her. When I disrupted her week, probably everything else she encountered amplified an edge of irritation in her. Neurophysiologically, her general arousal levels went up and lacking a good self-regulatory figure, her self-harm could be understood as her unhealthy attempt at self-regulation. If you cannot see what I mean about disruptions, just think of having a quarrel with a close friend or partner and think about how that can affect your day at work!

Now what comes to mind is a nine-year-old girl, Charlotte, who had been in therapy longer than Amal. The day after I completely misunderstood my importance to Charlotte and hadn't looked at how her rejection of me was linked to this feeling of being dropped by me she told me this dream: "I had a dream that a baby was falling off a cliff. Then I realized I had some life-saving equipment, and I was able to rescue the baby." Then she added, "I think the dream is because I felt bad because you didn't understand me yesterday."

The dream of the patient is where the meaning of the patient's life is located. Dreams, accompanying the child's awake behaviour, usually give the truest picture of the young person's interior world. Now we could look together and explore how we might comprehend her 'imprisoned self', for which she now had the psychological equipment of symbolizing feelings in dreams which she was willing to share with me. In this case it appeared that she was worried that getting better would mean ending therapy, and yet it was also true that she was beginning to be able to take some more responsibility for thinking about her infantile self. She felt dropped by me, but could try to talk about this feeling with me.

Remaining connected

> I feel fat and ugly. I don't deserve to have any pleasure. I pull away if you say anything good to me, I don't know why. I do not like myself. I feel I do not want to exist. I had a dream that I did not exist. I am confused. I can't remember. I don't know.

These are all statements made by Amal in the course of her psychotherapy. Such remarks generally reflect the young person's fragile internal psychic structure: internal parents whose understanding role in containing the child's feelings and conflicts is inadequate and damaged. The internal mother and the internal father are not resilient and need to be repaired. The young person feels fat because she has no boundaries around her feelings ... they are out of control. Her sense of ugliness is increased by the ugly hostile feelings projected into her internalized and external parents. In the process of thinking about the relationship with the psychotherapist I believe it is important to allow the therapist's and the child's feelings to flow freely. We cannot choose what we feel, but we can respond to the feelings we have, think about these feelings, and choose how we act in response to them.

Figures 8.4 and 8.5 show pictures drawn by 13-year-old anorectic girls in therapy.

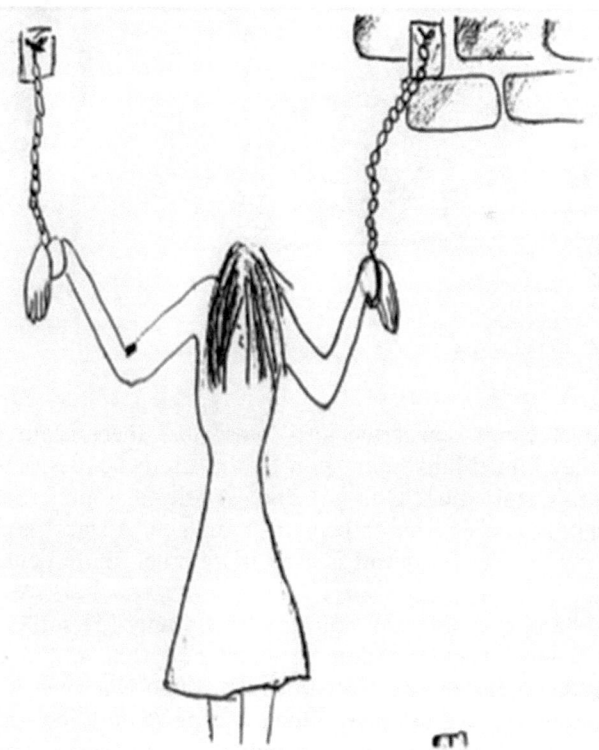

Figure 8.4 Hung on the cross

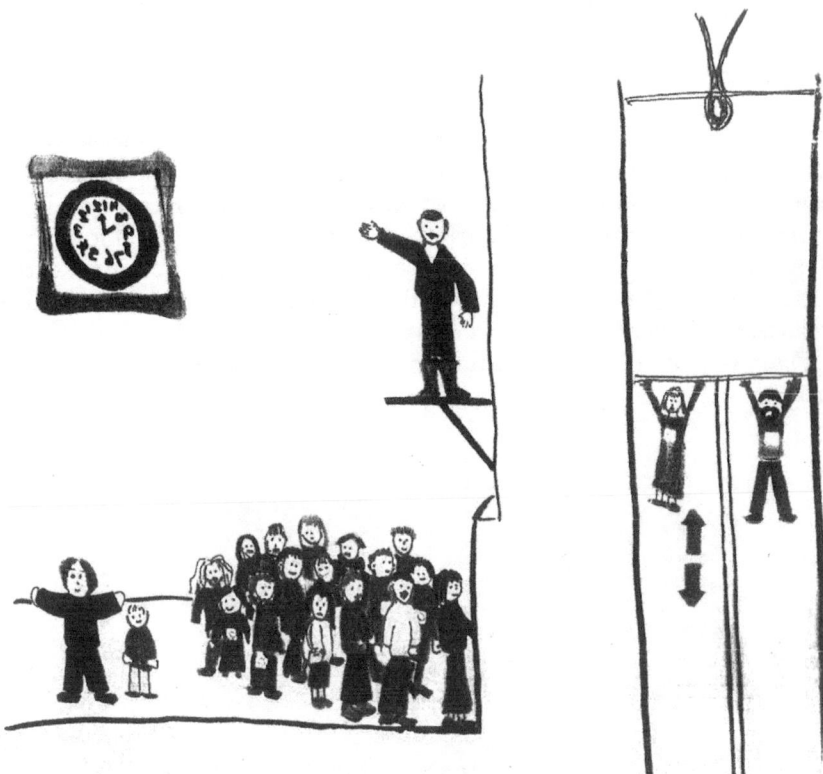

Figure 8.5 Hitler dictating destruction

Both these drawings depict the girls' sense that there is no freedom of choice, that they forced into submission by the anorectic, destructive part of the self dictating starvation. One girl said, 'Anorexia is preferable to being healthy though, because having to be perfect and get "A stars" is even worse.' Indeed her voice of perfectionism is even more cruel, more demanding and more difficult to please.

In psychotherapy I attempt to bear the young person's unbearable anxiety and fear of fragmentation. I understand that at the moment of anxiety, just like at the moment of drowning, there is a need to hold onto something, anything, to stay alive. When fearing dissolution, confusion or the craziness of psychotic states of mind, the young person grasps anything to survive. The 'anything' to which the young person adhesively clings may be:

- The anorectic voices dictating starving, exercising and vomiting.
- The self-harm thoughts promising salvation from psychic pain, loss of identity and psychotic confusion.
- The cruel, harsh superego dictating perfectionism.
- The sadomasochistic perverse and erotic phantasies providing excitement.
- The 'non-thinking apparatus' substituting denial, denudation of emotional life for truly knowing what one feels and thinks.

In *Attachment to the False Object* (1990), Barbara Segal and I explored the notion that one can help a young person to remain connected to the psychotherapist, to the helpful thoughts that arise in the session and to the a supportive figure outside the therapy. I say to even the most ill patients:

> At the moment when the self-harm thoughts, the anorectic thoughts, the perfectionistic thoughts present themselves to you, you often have a choice: You can choose to listen to them, follow their advice, lend them power by turning to them, and submitting to them or you can struggle to find your mother or father, your keyworker, a friend, your diary, the thoughts we have shared together and hold onto the life-raft we have created to hold you through these stormy moments of loneliness and separation from me.

I also suggest, 'It is possible to have some meaningful dialogue with the voices that are bullying you. You can ask them to leave you alone. You need support not cruel voices!'

At times the young person feels too identified with the cruel voices to do much until we think more about their cruelty. At other times, she has enough capacity to argue with them to leave her alone.

I believe that the young person is somehow aware as to whether or not the psychotherapist holds her in mind outside the psychotherapy hour – much as she might hold her family in mind.

The omnipotent destructive self attacks the young person who is trying to maintain a hope that holding onto the life-raft of therapy will eventually be helpful. In younger children, holding onto the hope that the therapist can be helpful is often symbolized by the presence of a boat and a bird in their drawings. The bird and boat suggest something about trust in the holding, thoughtful presence of the therapist. This suggests an introjection of an understanding therapist, which enables development of an inner security which permits the external therapist to have the freedom to come and go. It also implies sufficient love for the therapist and Self to tolerate separation and ambivalence when the therapist doesn't really adequately understand her.

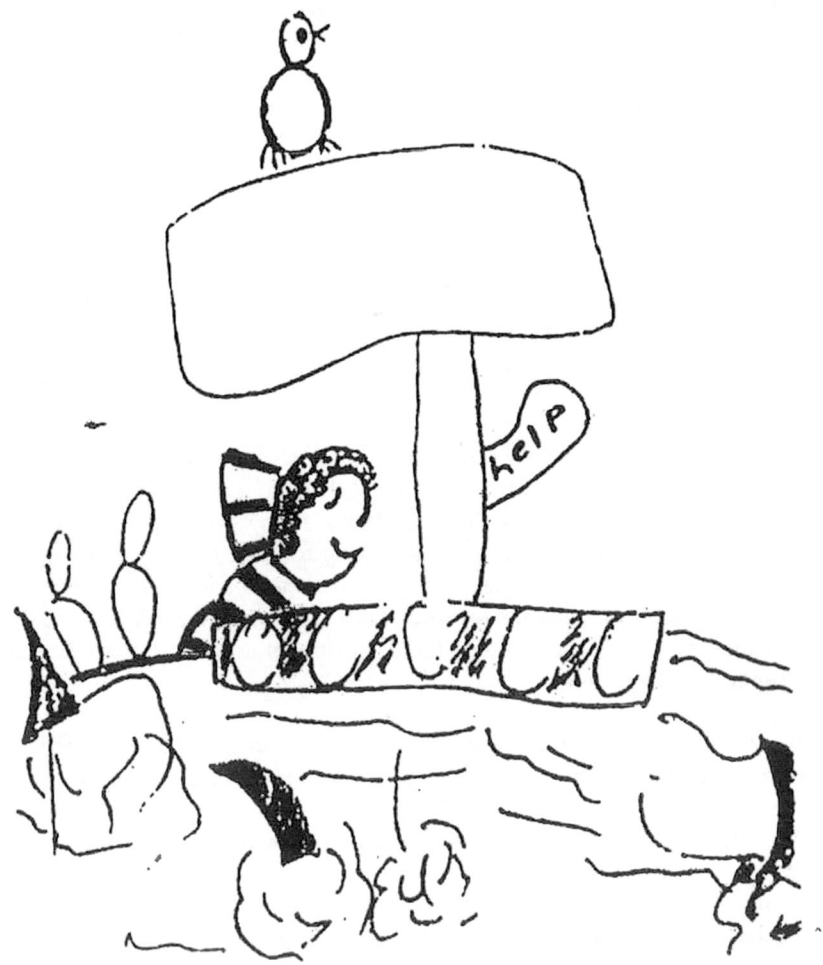

Figure 8.6 The boat with the bird nearby

An eating and sleep disordered 16-year-old Nigerian boy, Maceo, brought dreams reflecting his relationship with me at times of separation. One of his typical initial dreams was:

> There was a girl on the street with high volume music emanating from her Walkman radio. Maceo wanted to smash the machine, to smash her, she was a horrible dirty person, a prostitute. He wanted to go around the city cutting the wires of all Walkman radios. His association was that he wanted to throw hand-grenades at all the cars speeding by him on the road.

Here one sees that Maceo, being very possessive, had attacked me for being separate from him, attacked me for having a night-life with the father. I am experienced as a prostitute, dirtied by the oedipal coupling with the father, and he cuts the link with me.

Near the end of therapy Maceo began talking about his grandmother, whom he now realized he loved dearly. He said she mentioned something extremely painful to him just before she died: she had told him that she did not like how he was and she felt he did not love her. Maceo cried thinking about how terrible he really was at times.

One of his new experiences was feeling sadness rather than anger in facing separations. A dream, typical of those later in the therapy, was:

> Maceo was saying goodbye to a group of his best friends. They were giving presents to one another. He enjoyed his presents because he felt that people had actually thought about what they had chosen to give to him. He was so touched by their thoughtfulness that he was crying. He thought that when they were separated, reminding themselves of their friendship would make them feel sad.

In his therapy Maceo has now had a dream in which he is able to hold on to, and appreciate, my thoughtfulness and perhaps he has internalized our joint thoughtfulness about his emotional life, which includes his sadness about separating.

Conclusion

So, finally, let me return to my original question: 'Why do I do this psychotherapeutic work, with anorectic patients, that involves so much rejection of me?' Like little Jane, the infant described, and like Amal, the young person described, I too have faced rejection by my mother. Just prior to my birth she lost her first child. Like Jane and Amal, I have taken care of part of my infantile personality through primitive omnipotence, omniscience, denial. There still remains a very dependent part of myself, barricaded by books and knowledge about anorexia, barricaded through the use of professional achievement, barricaded through rejection of intimacy from myself and significant others, masking my infantile helplessness and dependence. I recognize that I 'freeze' to cover my emotions when I fear that my emotional needs cannot be fully met, either by me or significant others. In particular, that hostility towards the 'rejecting other', leads me to encapsulate parts of my feeling Self, and thus I lose access to this Self.

Now I can use the emotional understanding gained through preparing this chapter to either to defensively armour my Self more fully, to attempt to motivate, cure, and control the anorectic Amal, or to integrate this knowledge of my transference–countertransference experiences with anorectic young people into my personality and at the same time open my heart to the hate and love of Amal and all the other anorectic young people I see.

However, opening my heart to Amal means fully accepting Amal's dependence on my empathy, my understanding, my physical presence. I must fully acknowledge her fear, her hatred, her hostile or frightened turning away to her omnipotent structure, her self-starvation and self-harm which occurs when I have been unempathic, too intellectual, absent or too stupid to comprehend her.

Now in concluding this book representing the work of my lifetime, I see more clearly that I work as a psychotherapist to become more fully human, more integrated within myself; less hostile and more forgiving of rejection, and more loving and understanding in the face of hatred. I can utilize this greater self-knowledge to help others to feel known and understood. I hope you can too.

It is this really being there for Amal and sharing myself and being attuned with her that represents 'a different type of taming' of the solitary infantile Self. It is this acknowledgement of the dependency of the young person on the therapist – that unique therapist, as unique as the anorectic child's mother – which frees the infantile Self to be born into consciousness and integrated with the personality. It is this that fosters love and development within Amal's personality and mine.

References

Allen, J. and Fonagy, P. (Eds.) (2006). *Handbook of Mentalization-Based Treatment.* Chichester: John Wiley and Sons.

Alvarez, A. (1992). *Live Company. Psychoanalytic Psychotherapy with Autistic, Borderline, Deprived and Abused Children.* London and New York: Routledge.

Alvarez, A. (2012). Types of sexual transference and countertransference in psychotherapeutic work with adolescence. In: *The Thinking Heart.* London: Routledge, 116–138.

Alvarez, A. (2012). *The Thinking Heart.* London: Routledge.

Ambrosio, G. (Ed.) (2005). *On Incest: Psychoanalytic Perspectives.* London: Karnac.

Amez, S. and Botero, H. (2000). The mother, the baby, the pouch and the observer. Feeding difficulties of an infant on the kangaroo mother programme. *International Journal of Psychotherapy*, 3 (2): 33–45.

Balint, M. (1968). *The Basic Fault: Therapeutic Aspects of Regression.* Evanston: Northwestern University.

Barrett Browning, E. (1906). Grief. In: *The Poetical Works of Elizabeth Barrett Browning.* London: Smith, Elder, & Co.

Bateman, A. and Fonagy, P. (2004). *Psychotherapy for Borderline Personality Disorder.* Oxford: Oxford University Press.

Beck, A. T., Resnik, H. L. P. and Lettieri, D. (Eds.) (1974). *The Prediction of Suicide.* Bowie, Maryland: Charles Press Publishers.

Beebe, B. and Lachman, F. M. (1988). The contributions of mother-infant mutual influence to the origin of self and object representation. *Psychoanalytic Psychology*, 5 (4): 305–337.

Begoin, J. (2000). Love and destructivity from the aesthetic conflict to a revision of the concept of destructivity in the psyche. In M. Cohen and A. Hahn (Eds.), *Exploring the Work of Donald Meltzer.* London: Karnac.

Beresin, E. V., Gordon, C. and Herzog, D. B. (1989). The process of recovering from anorexia nervosa. *Journal of the American Academy of Psychoanalysis*, 17 (1): 103–130.

Bergman, N. (2014). www.kangaroomothercare.com. Article by Nils Bergman.

Bick, E. (1962). Child analysis today. *International Journal of Psychoanalysis*, 43: 328–332.

Bick, E. (1964). Notes on infant observation in psychoanalytic training. *International Journal of Psychoanalysis*, 45: 558–568.

Bick, E. (1968). The experience of skin in early object relations. *International Journal of Psychoanalysis*, 49: 484–486.

Bion, W. (1962). *Learning from Experience.* London: Heinemann.

Birksted-Breen, D. (1989). Working with an anorectic patient. *International Journal of Psychoanalysis*, 77: 29–40.

Bollas, C. (2000). *Hysteria*. London: Routledge.

Bourdouxhe, M. (1992). *La Femme De Gilles* (Trans. Faith Evans). Champaign, Illinois: Lime Tree Publications.

Bowlby, J. (1969). *Attachment and Loss, Vol. 1. Attachment*. London: Hogarth Press and Institute of Psycho-Analysis.

Bowlby, J. (1973). *Attachment and Loss, Vol. 2. Separation*. London: Hogarth Press and Institute of Psycho-Analysis.

Bowlby, J. (1980). *Attachment and Loss, Vol. 3. Loss*. London: Hogarth Press and Institute of Psycho-Analysis.

Box, S., Copley, B., Magagna, J. and Moustaki, M. (Eds.) (1981). *Psychotherapy with Families: An Analytic Approach*. London: Routledge.

Box, S., Copley, B., Magagna, J. and Moustaki, E. (Eds.) (2015). *Psychotherapy with Families*. London: Routledge.

Bozszormenyi-Nagy, I. and Spark, G. M. (1973). *Invisible Loyalties*. London: Harper and Row.

Branje, S. J. T. (2002). Relational support in families with adolescents. *Journal of Family Psychology*, 17: 445–459.

Brenman-Pick, I. (1985). Working through the counter-transference. *International Journal of Psychoanalysis*, 66: 157–166.

Briggs, A. (Ed.) (2002). *Surviving Space: Papers on Infant Observation*. London: Karnac.

Britton, R. (1989). The missing link: parental sexuality in the Oedipus complex. In: R. Britton, M. Feldman, E. O'Shaughnessy and J. Steiner (Eds.), *The Oedipus Complex Today*. London: Routledge, 34–45.

Bryant-Waugh, R. (1993). Overview of eating disorders. In: B. Lask and R. Bryant-Waugh, *Eating Disorders in Children*. Hove, England: Lawrence Erlbaum Associates.

Bryant-Waugh, R. and Kaminski, Z. (1993). Eating disorders in children: An overview. In B. Lask and R. Bryant-Waugh (Eds.), *Childhood Onset Anorexia Nervosa and Related Eating Disorders*. Hove: Lawrence Erlbaum Associates.

Bryant-Waugh, R., Knibbs, J., Fosson, A., Kaminski, Z. and Lask, B. (1988). Long term follow-up of patients with early onset anorexia nervosa. *Archives of Disease in Childhood*, 63: 5–9.

Buck, R. (1994). The neuropsychology of communication: spontaneous and symbolic aspects. *Journal of Pragmatics*, 22: 265–278.

Burgner, M. (1985). The oedipal experience: effects on development of an absent father. *International Journal of Psychoanalysis*, 66: 311–320.

Byng-Hall, J. (1980). The symptom bearer as marital distance regulator: clinical implications. *Family Process*, 19: 355–365.

Cameron, J. (1996). *The Vein of Gold: A Journey to your Creative Heart*. New York: Putnam & Sons.

Campbell, D. (1995). The role of the father in a pre-suicide state. *International Journal of Psychoanalysis*, 76: 315–323.

Campbell, D. and Hale, R. (1991). Suicidal acts. In: Holmes, J. (Ed.), *Textbook of Psychotherapy in Psychiatric Practice*. London: Longman Group.

Campbell, D. and Hale, R. (2017). *Working in the Dark*. London and New York: Routledge.

Casement, P. (1985). *On Learning from the Patient*. London: Tavistock Publications.

Chiland, C. (1982). A new look at fathers. *Psychoanalytic Study of the Child*, 37: 367–379.

Cooper, H. and Magagna, J. (2005). The development of self-esteem in infancy. In J. Magagna, N. Bakalar, H. Cooper, J. Levy, C. Norman and C. Shank (Eds.), *Intimate Transformations: Babies with their Families*. London: Karnac.

Cox, M. (1999). *Remorse and Reparation*. London: Jessica Kingsley.

Cozolino, L. J. (2006). The neuroscience of human relationships. In: Wilkinson, M. (Ed.), *Changing Minds in Therapy*. London and New York: W. W. Norton.

Crowe Ransom, J. (1991). In winter remembered. In: *Carcanet Selected Poems*. Manchester, UK: Carcanet Press.

Dare, C. (1993). The starving and the greedy: inner and outer objects in anorexia nervosa. *Journal of Child Psychotherapy*, 19 (2): 3–22.

Dare, C. and Crowther, C. (1995). Psychodynamic models of eating disorders. In: G. Szmukler, C. Dare and J. Treasure (Eds.), *Handbook of Eating Disorders: Theory, Treatment, and Research*. Chichester: Wiley.

Dare, C. and Eisler, I. (1995). Family therapy. In: G. Szmukler, C. Dare and J. Treasure (Eds.), *Handbook of Eating Disorders: Theory, Treatment, and Research*. Chichester: Wiley.

Dartington, A. and Magagna, J. (1994). Making a space for parents. In: S. Bow, B. Copley, J. Magagna and E. Moustaki-Smilansky (Eds.), *Crises in Adolescence*. London: Jason Aronson.

Dickinson, E. (1861). Nobody. In: T. H. Johnson (Ed.), *The Complete Poems of Emily Dickinson*. London: Faber and Faber Limited.

Dickinson, E. (1862). After great pain. In: T. H. Johnson (Ed.), *The Complete Poems of Emily Dickinson*. New York: Little, Brown and Company.

Dodd, V. (2004). Implications of kangaroo care for growth and development in preterm infants. *Journal of Obstetrics, Gynecology and Neonatal Nursing*, 34 (2): 218–232.

Doidge, N. (2007). *The Brain That Changes Itself*. London: Penguin Books Ltd.

Dominguez, G. and Magagna, J. (2009). The influence of conjoined twins on each other. In: V. Lewin and B. Sharp (Eds.), *The Sibling Relationship*. London: Karnac.

Dosamantes, I. (1992). The intersubjective relationship between therapist and patient: a key to understanding denied and denigrated aspects of the patient's self. *The Arts and Psychotherapy*, 19: 359–365.

Dubinsky, H. (2004). An anorectic girl's relationship to a very damaged persecutory internal object and its impact on her illness. In: G. Williams *et al.* (Eds.), *Generosity of Acceptance*. London: Karnac.

Eccleston, C. (2019). *I Love the Bones of You*. London: Simon and Schuster.

Emanuel, R. (2001). A-void: an exploration of defences against sensing nothingness. *International Journal of Psychoanalysis*, 82: 1063–1084.

Ermann, G. and Lazar, R. A. (2002). From dyad to triad: Observations on the similarities and differences in the roles and functions of mother and father in infantile development. *The International Journal of Infant Observation*, 5 (3): 83–100.

Farmer, S. and Hirsch, S. (1979). *The Suicide Syndrome*. Cambridge, England: Cambridge University Press.

Farrell, E. (1995). *Lost for Words: The Psychoanalysis of Anorexia and Bulimia*. London: Process Press.

Fast, I. (1979). Developments in gender identity: gender differentiation in girls. *International Journal of Psychoanalysis*, 60: 443–453.

Favazza, A. R. (1998). *Bodies under Siege: Self-mutilation and Body Modification in Culture and Psychiatry*. Baltimore, Maryland: John Hopkins.

Fenichel, O. (1945). *Anorexia*. In: H. Fenichel (Ed.), *The Collected Papers of Otto Fenichel*. New York: Norton, 296–304.

Fonagy, P., Gergerly, G., Jurist, E. and Target, M. (2004). *Affect Regulation, Mentalization, and the Development of the Self*. London: Karnac.

Fonagy, P., Steele, M., Moran, G. S., Steele, H. and Higgitt, A. (1993). Measuring the ghost in the nursery. An empirical study of the relation between parents' mental representation of childhood experiences and their infants' security of attachment. *Infant Mental Health Journal*, 33: 200–217.

Fonagy, P. and Target, M. (1997). Attachment and reflective function. *Development and Psychopathology*, 9: 679–700.

Fosson, A., Knibbs, J., Bryant-Waugh, R. and Lask, B. (1987). Early onset anorexia nervosa, *Archives of Disease in Childhood*, 62: 114–118.

Fraiberg, S., Adelson, E. and Shapiro, V. (1980). Ghosts in the nursery: a psychoanalytic approach to impaired infant-mother relationships. In: S. Fraiberg (Eds.), *Clinical Studies in Infant Mental Health*. London: Tavistock, 164–193.

Freud, S. (1911). Handling of dream interpretation in psychoanalysis. *S.E. 12*. London: Hogarth Press and Institute of Psychoanalysis.

Freud, S. (1931). Female sexuality. *S.E. 21*. London: Hogarth Press and Institute of Psychoanalysis.

Gammill, J. (1980). Some reflections on analytic listening and the dream screen. *International Journal of Psychoanalysis*, 61 (3): 275–381.

Garber, J. and Seligman, M. (Eds.) (1980). *Human Helplessness: Theory and Application*. New York and London: Academic Press.

García-Villamisar, D., Dattilo, J. and Del Pozo, A. (2012). Depressive mood, eating disorder symptoms, and perfectionism in female college students: a mediation analysis. *Eating Disorders*, 20 (1): 60–72.

Gardener, F. (2001). *Self Harm*. Hove and New York: Brunner and Routledge.

Garland, C. (1999). *Understanding Trauma: A Psychoanalytic Approach*. London: Duckworth.

Garner, D. and Garfinkel, P. (Eds.) (1997). *Handbook of Treatment for Eating Disorders* (2nd edition). London: Guildford Press.

Geller, J., Cockel, S. J. and Drab, D. L. (2001). Assessing readiness for change in eating disorders: the psychosomatic properties of the readiness and motivation interview. *Psychological Assessment*, 13: 189–198.

Gibran, K. (1933). On Children. In: *Garden of the Prophet*. New York: Knopf.

Gluckman, C. (1987). Incest in psychic reality. *Journal of Child Psychotherapy*, 13 (1): 109–123.

Goldberg, S. (1979). Premature Birth: consequences for the parent-infant relationship: the normal pattern of interaction in which both infant and parent initiate and respond to mutually complementary behavior is difficult to establish when the infant is premature. *American Scientist*, 67 (2): 214–220.

Goldman, E. and Morrison, D. (1984). *Psychodrama: Experience and Process*. Dubique, IA: Kendall-Hunt.

Goodsitt, A. (1997). Eating disorders: A self-psychological perspective. In D. Garner and P. Garfinkel (Eds.), *Handbook of Treatment for Eating Disorders* (2nd ed.). London: Guilford Press.

Goretta, C. (1977). The Lacemaker. A film based on the novel by P. Laine (1974), *Le Dentelliere*. Gallimand.

Graham, P. (1986). *Child Psychiatry: A Developmental Approach*. Oxford: Oxford University Press.

Gray, G. E. (1983). Severe depression: A patient's thoughts. *British Journal of Psychiatry*, 143: 319–322.

Greatrex, T. S. (2002). Projective identification: how does it work? *Neuropsychoanalysis*, 4: 87–197.

Green, A. H. (1978). Psychopathology of abused children. *Journal of the American Academy of Child Psychiatry*, 17: 92–100.

Hadiks, D. (1994). Nonverbal aspects of therapist attunement. *Journal of Clinical Psychology*, 50: 393–405.

Haim, A. (1970). *Adolescent Suicide*. London: Tavistock Publications.

Hale, R. and Campbell, D. (1991). Suicidal acts. In: J. Holmes (Ed.), *Textbook of Psychotherapy in Psychiatric Practice*, 287–306. Edinburgh: Churchill Livingston.

Harrison, K. (2003). Mother's Day card. In: *Seeking Rapture*. New York: Random House/Routledge.

Hinshelwood, R. (1994). *Clinical Klein*. London: Free Association Books.

Isaacs, S. (1948). The nature and function of phantasy. *International Journal of Psychoanalysis*, 29: 73–97.

Jacobs, T. J. (2005). Discussion. In B. Beebe, S. Knoblauch, J. Rustin and D. Sorter (Eds.), *Forms of Intersubjectivity in Infant Research and Adult Treatment*. New York: Other Press.

Janssen, P. (1994). *Psychoanalytic Therapy in the Hospital Setting*. London: Routledge.

Javanbakht, A. and Ragan, C. J. (2008). A neural network model for transference and repetition compulsion based on pattern completion. *Journal of the American Academy of Psychoanalysis and Dynamic Psychiatry*, 36 (2): 255–278.

Jools, P. (1991). Some thoughts on twin psychotherapy. *Australian Journal of Psychotherapy* 10 (2): 180–192.

Jordon, M. and Johnson, S. (2009). Personal communication.

Joseph, B. (1985). Transference: the total situation . *International Journal of Psychoanalysis*, 59: 223–228.

Kandel, E. R. (2006). *In Search of Memory*. New York: W.W. Norton & Co.

Kaplan-Solms, K. and Solms, M. (2002). *Clinical Studies in Neuro-psychoanalysis*. New York: Karnac.

Kennedy, R. and Magagna, J. (1994). The aftermath of murder. In S. Box, R. Copley, J. Magagna and E. Moustaki-Smilansky (Eds.), *Crisis at Adolescence*, 203–221. London: Jason Aronson.

Kestenbaum, C. J. and Stone, M. H. (1976). The effects of fatherless homes upon daughters: clinical impressions regarding paternal deprivation. *Journal of the American Academy of Psychoanalysis*, 4 (2): 171–190.

Klein, M. (1937). Love, guilt and reparation. In: *Vol. 1: Love, Guilt and Reparation and Other Works 1921–1945*. London: Hogarth. 1975.

Klein, M. (1945). The Oedipus complex in the light of early anxieties. In: *Vol. 1: Love, Guilt and Reparation and Other Works 1921–1945*. London: Hogarth. 1975.

Klein, M. (1946). Notes on some schizoid mechanisms. *International Journal of Psychoanalysis*, 27: 99–100.

Klein, M. (1963). On the sense of loneliness. In: *Envy and Gratitude and Other Works*. Reprinted 1980. London: Hogarth, 300–313.

Klein, S. (1980). Autistic phenomena in neurotic patients. *International Journal of Psychoanalysis*, 31: 108–116.

Kohut, H. (1971). *The Analysis of the Self*. New York: International Universities Press.

Krystal, H. (1978). Trauma and affects. *Psychoanalytic Study of the Child*, 33: 81–116.

Kumari, V. (2006). Do psychotherapies produce neurobiological effects? *Acta Neuro-Psychiatrica*, 18 (2): 61–70.

Lask, B. (1993). Management overview. In: B. Lask and R. Bryant-Waugh (Eds.), *Childhood Onset Anorexia Nervosa and Related Eating Disorders*. London: Lawrence Erlbaum.

Lask, B. (2012). The sound of silence. *In:* J. Magagna *(Ed.), The Silent Child: Communication Without Words*. London: Karnac.

Lask, B. and Bryant-Waugh, R. (1993). *Childhood Onset Anorexia Nervosa and Related Eating Disorders* (2nd ed.). London: Psychology Press.

Lask, B., Britten, C., Kroll, L., Magagna, J. and Tranter, M. (1991). Pervasive refusal. *Archives of Diseases in Childhood*, 66: 966–990.

Lask, B., Nunn, K. and Owen, I. (2013). Pervasive refusal syndrome (PRS) 21 years on: A reconceptualisation and a renaming. *European Child and Adolescent Psychiatry*, 23 (3).

Laufer, M. E. (1981). The adolescent's use of the body in object relationships and in the transference – a comparison of borderline and narcissistic modes of functioning. *Psychoanalytic Study of the Child*, 36: 163–180.

Laufer, M. (1989). Adolescent sexuality – a body/mind continuum. *Psychoanalytic Study of the Child*, 44: 281–294.

Laufer, M. (Ed.) (1995). *The Suicidal Adolescent*. London: Karnac.

Lawn, J., Mwansa-Kambafwile, J., Horta, B.L., Fernando, C., Barros, F.C. and Cousens, C. (2011). Kangaroo mother care' to prevent neonatal deaths due to preterm birth complications. *International Journal of Epidemiology*, 40 (2): 525–528.

Lawrence, M. (2001). Loving them to death: The anorexic and her objects . *International Journal of Psychoanalysis*, 82: 43–45.

Le Grange, D., Eisler, I., Dare, C. and Hodes, M. (1992). Family criticism and self-starvation: a study of expressed emotion. *Journal of Family Therapy*, 14: 177–192.

Leff, J. and Vaughan, C. (1983). *Expressed Emotion in Families*. New York: Guilford Press.

Leonard, M. R. (1966). Fathers and daughters – the significance of 'fathering' in the psychosexual development of the girl. *International Journal of Psychoanalysis*, 47: 325–334.

Leunig, M. (1990). *A Common Prayer*. North Blackburn, Victoria, Australia: Collins Dove.

Levin, F. M. (1980). Metaphor, affect and arousal: how interpretations might work. *Annual of Psychoanalysis*, 8: 231–245.

Lewin, V. (2004). *The Twin in the Transference*. London and Philadelphia: Whurr.

Lewis, P. P. (1992). The creative arts in transference/countertransference relationships. *The Arts in Psychotherapy*, 19: 317–323.

Lewis, H. L. and MacGuire, M. P. (1985). Review of a group for parents of anorexics. *Journal of Psychiatric Research*, 19, 453–458.

Likierman, M. (1997). On rejection: adolescent girls and anorexia. *Journal of Child Psychotherapy*, 23 (1): 61–80.

Limperopoulos, C., Bassan, H., Sullivan, N. R., Soul, J. S., Robertson, R. Jr., Moore, M., Ringer, S., Volpe, J. and du Plessis, A. J. (2008). Positive screening for autism in expreterm infants: prevalence and risk factors. *Pediatrics*. April 2008, 121 (4): 758–765.

Linden, D. E. J. (2006). How psychotherapy changes the brain: the contribution of functional neuro-imaging and psychotherapy. *Molecular Psychiatry*, 11: 528–538.

Litman, R. E. (1980). The dream in the suicidal situation. In: J. M. Natterson (Ed.), *The Dream in Clinical Practice*. New York: Aronson.

Lock, J. and Le Grange, D. (2015). *Treatment Manual for Anorexia Nervosa, Second Edition: A Family-Based Approach*. New York: Guildford Press.

Lord, M. M. and Stone, C. (1973). Fathers and daughters: a study of three poems. *Contemporary Psychoanalysis*, 9 (2): 526–539.

Lubbe, T. (2003). *The Borderline Psychotic Child*. London: Routledge.

MacLeod, S. (1982). *The Art of Starvation: A Story of Anorexia and Survival* London: Schocken Books.

Magagna, J. (1987). Three years of infant observation with Mrs. Bick. *Journal of Child Psychotherapy*, 13 (1): 19–39.

Magagna, J. (1988). Working with a 14-year-old and a wrecked girl. In: I. Rossi, S. Bastianelli*et al.* (Eds.), *Counselling Approccio Clinico in Adolescenza*. Bologna: Cooperativa Libraria University Editrice.

Magagna, J. (1994). Attacks on life. In: M. Rustin and E. Quagliata (Eds.), *Assessment in Psychotherapy*. London: Karnac.

Magagna, J. (1996). *Understanding the Unspoken: Psychotherapy with Children Having Severe Eating Disorders, in Psychosomatic Problems in Children* (ACPP Occasional Papers No. 12), London.

Magagna, J. (1998). Psychodynamic psychotherapy in an in-patient setting. In: J. Greene and B. Jacobs (Eds.), *The Child Psychiatry In-Patient Unit*, London: Routledge.

Magagna, J. (2000). Individual psychotherapy. In: B. Lask and R. Bryant-Waugh, (Eds.) *Anorexia Nervosa and Related Eating Disorders in Childhood and Adolescence* (second edition). London: Psychology Press.

Magagna, J. (2002). Mrs. Bick's contribution to the understanding of severe feeding difficulties and pervasive refusal. In. A. Briggs (Ed.), *Surviving Space: Papers on Infant Observation*. London: Karnac.

Magagna, J. (2004). Transformation from twin to individual. In: V. Lewin and B. Sharp (Eds.), *Siblings in Development*. London and Philadelphia: Whurr.

Magagna, J. (2007). Transformation. From twin to individual. *Journal of Child Psychotherapy*, 33 (1): 51–69.

Magagna, J. (2005). The reparative aspects of the dreams of children (La valutazione dei tentative di riparazione nei sogni dei bambini). In: M. Camoni*et al.* (Eds.), *Sogni*. Pisa: Editioni ETS.

Magagna, J. (2012). *The Silent Child: Communication without Words*. London: Karnac.

Magagna, J., Bakalar, N., Cooper, H., Levy, J., Norman, C. and Shank, C. (2005). *Intimate Transformations: Babies with their Families*. London: Karnac.

Magagna, J. and Owen, I. (2011). Svezzarsi dal gemello piu forte: un ppunto di vista neuro-psicoanalitico. In: C. Busato and M. Mondello (Eds.), *Nuovi assetti della clinicaa in eta evolutive*. Quaderni di Psicoterapia Infantile.

Magagna, J. and Piercey, J. (2020). Collaborative work with parents. *British Journal of Psychotherapy*, 36 (2): 275–286.

Magagna, J. and Segal, B. (1990). L'attachment et les procesus psychotiques chez une adolescent anorexique. *Psychoses et Creation, L'Ecole Anglais.* Groupe de recherché et d'application des concepts psychoanalystiques a la psychoses (Eds.). Paris: Diffusion Navarin/Seuil.

Malan, D. H. (1997). *Anorexia, Murder and Suicide.* Oxford, England: Reed Educational and Professional Publishing Ltd.

Malouf, D. (1999). *An Imaginary Life.* London: Vintage Press.

Mancia, M. (2005). Implicit memory and the early repressed unconscious. *International Journal of Psychoanalysis,* 87: 83–101.

Matthews, P. (1988). Where beauty lies. In: J. Ramsay (Ed.), *Transformation: The Poetry of Spiritual Consciousness.* London: Rivelin Graphen.

Meltzer, D. (1967). *The Psychoanalytic Process.* London: Heinemann.

Meltzer, D. (1973). *Sexual States of Mind.* Perthshire: Clunie Press.

Meltzer, D. (1984). *Dreamlife: A Re-examination of Psychoanalytic Theory and Technique.* Perthshire: Clunie Press.

Meltzer, D. (1986). *Studies in Extended Metapsychology.* Perthshire: Clunie Press.

Meltzer, D. (1992). *The Claustrum.* Perthshire: Clunie Press.

Meltzer, D. (1994). Temperature and distance as a technical dimension of interpretation. In: A. Hahn (Ed.), *Sincerity and Other Works.* London: Karnac.

Michati Squittieri, L. (1999). Problems of female sexuality: the defensive function of certain phantasies about the body. *International Journal of Psychoanalysis,* 80: 645–660.

Miller, M. L. (2008). The emotionally engaged analyst. 1. Theories of affect and their influence on therapeutic action. *Psychoanalytic Psychology,* 25 (1): 3–25.

Mind (2017). Newsletter. April 12, 2017.

Minuchin, S., Rosman, B. and Baker, L. (1978). *Psychosomatic Families.* Cambridge, MA: Harvard University Press.

Money-Kyrle, R. (1978). Normal counter-transference and some of its deviations. In: Meltzer, D. and O'Shaughnessy, E. (Eds.), *The Collected Papers of Roger Money-Kyrle,* 330–342. Perthshire: Clunie (Original work published 1956).

Natterson, J. (1980). *The Dream in Clinical Practice.* New York: Jason Aronson.

Nelson, E., Leibenlluft, E., McClure, E. and Pine, D. (2005). The social re-orientation of adolescence: a neuroscience perspective on the process and its relation to psychopathology. *Psychological Medicine,* 35: 163–174.

Neubauer, P. B. (1960). The one-parent child and his oedipal development. *Psychoanalytic Study of the Child,* 15: 286–309.

National Institute of Health and Care Excellence (NICE) (2018). 21 September 2018 on www.nice.org.uk/guidance/qs175.

Nunn, K. and Thompson, L. (1996). The pervasive refusal syndrome: learned helplessness and hopelessness. *Clinical Child Psychology and Psychiatry,* 1: 121–132.

Nunn, K. P., Lask, B. and Owen, I. (2014). Pervasive refusal syndrome (PRS) 21 years on: a re-conceptualisation and a renaming. *European Child & Adolescent Psychiatry,* 23 (3): 163–172.

Orbach, S. (1994). Working with the false body. In: A. Erskine and D. Judd (Eds.), *The Imaginative Body.* London: Whurr.

O'Shaughnessy, E. (1964). The absent object. *Journal of Child Psychotherapy,* 1 (2): 34–43.

Padel, J. H. (1987). *The Oxford Companion to the Mind.* Oxford: Oxford University Press.

Palazzoli, M. S. (1978). *Self-Starvation: From Individual to Family Therapy in the Treatment of Anorexia Nervosa*. New York: Jason Aronson.

Pally, R. (2000). *The Mind-Brain Relationship*. London and New York: Karnac.

Palmer, R. L., Oppenheimer, R., Dignon, A., Chaloner, D. A. and Howells, K. (1990) Childhood sexual experiences with adults reported by women with eating disorders: an extended series. *British Journal of Psychiatry*, 156: 699–703.

Panksepp, J. and Bernatzky, G. (2002). Emotional sounds and the brain: The neuro-affective foundations of musical appreciation. *Behavioral Processes*, 60: 133–155.

Parker, R. (2009). *Body Image*. Unpublished manuscript.

Pedersen, C. A. (2004). Biological aspects of social bonding and the roots of human violence. *Annals of the New York Academy of Sciences*, 1036, 106–127.

Pessoa, F. (1917). *In The Surprise of Being*. Translated by J. Greene and C. de Azevedo Mafra (1986). London: Angel Books.

Petkova, H., Simic, M., Nicholls, D., Ford, T., Prina, A. M., Stuart, R., Livingstone, N., Kelly, G., Macdonald, G., Eisler, I., Gowers, S., Barrett, B. M. and Byford, S (2019). Incidence of anorexia nervosa in UK and Ireland: A national surveillance study. *British Medical Journal*, 9 (10).

Petrelli, D. (2003). Fantasies concerning body functioning in an anorectic adolescent. In: G. Williams, P. Williams, J. Desmarais, and K. Ravenscroft (Eds.), *Exploring Eating Disorders in Adolescents: The Generosity of Acceptance*, Vol. 2. London: Karnac.

Plath, S. (1981). Daddy. In: *Sylvia Plath: Collected Poems*. London: Faber and Faber.

Pocock, D. (1992). Parental perceptions of sibling differences: towards a theory of sibling differences. *Journal of Family Therapy*, 14 (2): 123–144.

Piontelli, A. (1989). A study on twins before and after birth. *International Review of Psychoanalysis*, 16: 413–426.

Piontelli, A. (1997). *From Fetus to Child*. London: Routledge.

Quagliata, E. (2002). *Un Bisogna Vitale*. Rome: Astrolabio.

Racker, H. (1968). *Transference and Countertransference*. London: Hogarth Press.

Ramachandran, V. S. and Blakeslee, S. (1998). *Phantoms in the Brain*. New York: William Morrow.

Randall, E. (1988). Beyond all other. In: J. Ramsay (Ed.), *Transformation: The Poetry of Spiritual Consciousness*. London: Rivelin Graphen.

Reich, T. (1948). *Listening with the Third Ear*. New York: Farrar, Jones, Giroux.

Reid, M. (2013). *Grief in the mother's eyes*. Unpublished talk given to the Washington Institute of Psychoanalysis, 5 April 2013, Washington DC.

Reid, M. (2014). Personal communication.

Rey, H. (1994). Anorexia nervosa. In: J. Magagna (Ed.), *Universals of Psychoanalysis*. London: Free Association Press.

Rilke, M. R. (1981). Unpublished poem. In: R. Britton, *Belief and Imagination* (1998: 157). Ed. and trans. M. Hamburger, *An Unofficial Rilke*. London: Anvil Poetry.

Ritvo, S. (1976). From adolescent to woman. *Journal of the American Psychoanalytic Association*, 24: 127–137.

Riviere, J. (1955). The unconscious phantasy of an inner world reflected in examples from literature. In: M. Klein, P. Heimann and R. E. Money-Kyrle (Eds.), *New Directions in Psychoanalysis*, 346–369. London: Tavistock Publications.

Robertson, J. and Robertson, J. (1971). Young children in brief separation: a fresh book. *Psychoanalytic Study of the Child*, 26: 264–315.

Rogeberg, K. (1990). Eating disorders and the family: experiences gathered in a parent support group. *Acta Psychiatrica Scandinavica*, 82: 50–51.

Rose, J. and Garfinkel, P. E. (1980). A parent's group in the management of anorexia nervosa. *Canadian Journal of Psychiatry*, 25: 228–233.

Rosenfeld, H. (1971). A clinical approach to the psychoanalytic theory of the life and death instincts: An investigation into the aggressive aspects of narcissism. *International Journal of Psychoanalysis*, 52: 169–178.

Rosenfeld, H. (1975). *Psychotic States*. London: Hogarth Press.

Rosenfeld, H. (1987a). *Impasse and Interpretation*. London: Tavistock Publications.

Rosenfeld, H. (1987b). Projective identification in clinical practice. In: *Impasse and Interpretation*, 157–190. London: Routledge.

Rosenfeld, D. (2012). *The Creation of the Self and Language*. London: Karnac.

Russell, G. (1985). Pre-menarcheal anorexia nervosa and its sequelae. *Journal of Psychiatric Research*, 19: 363–369.

Russell, G. F. M., Szmukler, G. I., Dare, C. and Eisler, I. (1987). An evaluation of family therapy in anorexia nervosa and bulimia nervosa. *Archives of General Psychiatry*, 44: 1047–1056.

Schore, A. N. (1994). *Affect Regulation and the Origin of the Self: The Neurobiology of Emotional Development*. Hillsdale, NJ: Lawrence Erlbaum Associates.

Schore, A. (2002). Clinical implications of a psychoneurobiological model of projective identification. In: S. Alhanati (Ed.), *Primitive Mental States, Volume II*. London: Karnac.

Schore, J. R. and Schore, A. N. (2008). Modern attachment theory: the central role of affect-regulation in development and treatment. *Clinical Social Work Journal*, 36: 9–20.

Schutzenberger, A. (1998). *The Ancestor Syndrome*. London and New York: Routledge.

Schwartz, J. M. and Begley, S. (2002). *The Mind and the Brain: Neuroplasticity and the Power of Mental Force*. New York: Regan Books/HarperCollins.

Segal, H. (1973). *Introduction to the Work of Melanie Klein*. London: Hogarth Press.

Segal, H. (1981). *The Work of Hanna Segal*. London: Jason Aronson.

Selekman, M. (2006). *Working with Self-Harming Adolescents*. New York: W.W. Norton and Company, Inc.

Sexton, A. (1981). *Complete Poems*. Boston: Houghton Mifflin Company.

Sgroi, S. (1982). *Handbook of Clinical Interventions in Child Sexual Abuse*. Lexington, Maine: Lexington Books.

Shapiro, R. L. (1967). The origin of adolescent disturbance in the family: some considerations in theory and implications for therapy. In: G. H. Zuk and I. Boszormenyi-Nagy (Eds.), *Family Therapy and Disturbed Families*. Palo Alto, CA: Science and Behavior Books.

Shelley, R. (1997). *Anorexics on Anorexia*. London: Jessica Kingsley.

Shneidman, E. S., Farberow, N. L. and Litman, R. E. (Eds.) (1976). *The Psychology of Suicide*. New York: Science House.

Shulman, S. and Seiffge-Krenke, I. (1997). *Fathers and Adolescents: Developmental and Clinical Perspectives*. London: Routledge.

Simon, P. and Garfunkel, A. (1964). *The Sound of Silence*. Columbia Records, Catalogue number 4–43396.

Simpson, M. A. (1976). Self-mutilation. *British Journal of Hospital Medicine*, 16: 430–438.

Slade, A. (2007). Reflective parenting programs: theory and development. *Psychoanalytic Inquiry*, 26 (4): 640–657.

Sohn, L. (1985). Anorexic and bulimic states of mind in the psycho-analytic treatment of anorexic/bulimic patients and psychotic patients. *Psychoanalytic Psychotherapy*, 1: 49–56.

Spitz, R. A. (1955). The primal cavity: a contribution to the genesis of perception and its role for psychoanalytical theory. *Psychoanalytic Study of the Child*, 10: 215–240.

Spitz, R. (1965). *The First Year of Life*. New York: International Universities Press.

St. Exupery, A. (1995). *The Little Prince*. London: Mammoth Press.

Stein, A. (1994). *Formerly Anorectic Mothers and Their Young Children* (Videotapes). London: Tavistock Clinic.

Stein, D. J. and Vythilingum, B. (2009). Love and attachment: the psychobiology of social bonding. *CNS Spectrums*, 14 (5): 239–242.

Steiner, J. (1993). *Psychic Retreats*. London: Tavistock/Routledge.

Stern, D. N. (1985). *The Interpersonal World of the Infant: A View from Psychoanalysis and Developmental Psychology*. New York: Basic Books.

Stoller, R. (1991). *Pain and Passion: A Psychoanalyst Explores the World of Sadomasochism*. New York: Plenum Press.

Symington, J. (1985). The establishment of female genitality. *Free Associations*, 1: 57–85.

Symington, J. (2002). Mrs. Bick and infant observation. In: Briggs, A. (Ed.), *Surviving Space: Papers on Infant Observation*. London: Karnac.

Szmukler, G., Dare, C., and Treasure, J. (1995). *Handbook of Eating Disorders: Theory, Treatment, and Research*. Chichester: Wiley.

Tähkä, V. A. (1979). On some narcissitic aspects of self-destructive behaviour and their influence on its predictability. *Psychiatria Fennica*, 1978: 59–62.

Tann, J. (2005). *Can she really decide? An ethical approach to choice and compulsion in anorexia nervosa*. Presentation to the International Eating Disorder Conference in London.

Tereul, G. (1966). Considerations for a diagnosis in marital psychotherapy. *British Journal of Medical Psychology*, 39: 231.

Tessman, L. (1989). Fathers and daughters: early tones, later echoes. In: S. Cath, A. Gerwitt, and L. Gunsberg (Eds.), *Fathers and Their Families*. Hillsdale, NJ: The Analytic Press.

Trauffaut, F. (1975). L'Histoire d'Adele H. A film based on A. Hugo (1968), *Le Journal d'Adèle Hugo*. Paris: Lettres modernes.

Treasure, J. and Holland, A. J. (1989). Genetic vulnerability to eating disorders: evidence from twin and family studies. In: H. Remschmidt and M. H. Schmidt (Eds.), *Anorexia Nervosa*. Toronto: Hogrefe and Huber.

Trevarthan, C. (1980). The foundations of intersubjectivity; development of interpersonal and co-operative understanding in infants. In: D. R. Olson (Ed.), *Before Speech: The Beginning of Interpersonal Communication*. New York: Cambridge University Press.

Trowell, J. and Etchegoyan, A. (Eds.) (2002). *The Importance of Fathers*. London: Brunner-Routledge.

Tucker, C. (1983). Proximate effects of sexual abuse in childhood. *American Journal of Psychiatry*, 139: 1252–1256.

Turp, M. (2003). *Hidden Self-Harm*. London and Philadelphia: Jessica Kingsley Publishers.

Tustin, F. (1986). *Autistic Barriers in Neurotic Patients.* London: Karnac.

Vaughn, C. and Leff, J. P. (1985). *Expressed Emotion in Families: Its Significance for Mental Illness.* New York: Guilford Press.

Venzlaff, U. (1964). Mental disorders resulting from racial persecution outside concentration camps. *International Journal of Social Psychiatry*, 10: 177–183.

Vitousek, K. and Gray, J. (2005). Eating disorders. In: G. Gabbard, J. Beck and J. Holmes (Eds.), *Oxford Handbook of Psychotherapy.* Oxford: Oxford University Press.

Waddell, M. (1998). *Inside Lives: Psychoanalysis and the Growth of the Personality.* London: Karnac.

White, M. (1989). The externalising of the problem and the re-authoring of lives and relationships. *Dulwich Centre Newsletter*, 3–20.

White, R. (2004). Mothers' arms: the past and future locus of neonatal care. *Clinics in Perinatology*, June 2004, 2 (31): 293.

Williams, G., Williams, P., Ravenscroft, K. and Desmaris, J. H. (2004). *Generosity of Acceptance.* London: Karnac.

World Health Organisation (WHO) (2014). Found in: www.who.int/maternal_child_a dolescent/topics/newborn/care_of_pre-term/en. Accessed May 30, 2014.

Wilkinson, M. (2010). *Changing Minds in Therapy.* London and New York: W. W. Norton and Co.

Williams, D. (1992). *Nobody Nowhere.* Toronto, Ontario: Doubleday.

Williams, G. (1997). Reflections on some dynamics of eating disorders: 'no entry' defences and foreign bodies. *International Journal of Psychoanalysis*, 78: 927–941.

Winnicott, D. (1958). *Collected Papers: Through Paediatrics to Psycho-Analysis.* London: Tavistock Publications, 243–254.

Winnicott, D. W. (1963). The mentally ill in your caseload. *In: The Maturational Processes and the Facilitating Environment.* London: Hogarth Press, 1965.

Winnicott, D. W. (1964). *The Child, the Family and the Outside World.* London: Penguin.

Wisdom, J. O. (1976). The role of the father in the mind of parents, in psychoanalytic theory and in the life of the infant. *International Journal of Psychoanalysis*, 3: 231–239.

Wolpert, L. (1999). *Malignant Sadness.* London: Faber and Faber Limited.

Wren, B. and Lask, B. (1993). Aetiology. In: B. Lask and R. Bryant-Waugh (Eds.), *Childhood Onset Anorexia and Related Eating Disorders.* London: Lawrence Erlbaum Associates.

Wright, S. (2004). *Palatable Differences: An Exploration of the Development of Anorexia Nervosa within the Context of the Twin Relationship Experience.* Doctoral dissertation: University of East London.

Yeats, W. B. (2001). A prayer for old age. In: *Collected Work of W.B. Yeats.* New York: Simon and Schuster Inc.

Zinner, J. and Shapiro, R. (1972). Projective identification as a mode of perception and behaviour in families of adolescents. *International Journal of Psychoanalysis*, 53: 523–530.

Index